GUIDE FOR HOUSE PHYSICIANS
IN THE
NEUROLOGICAL UNIT

GUIDE FOR HOUSE PHYSICIANS IN THE NEUROLOGICAL UNIT

T. Fowler, D.M., F.R.C.P.

*Consultant Neurologist
The Brook Hospital, Woolwich, and
for the Dartford and Tunbridge Wells
Health Districts*

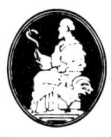

WILLIAM HEINEMANN MEDICAL BOOKS LTD.
LONDON

First published 1982

© T. Fowler 1982

ISBN 0-433-10688-3

Printed and bound in Great Britain by Henry Ling Ltd, Dorchester

PREFACE

This book is intended as a guide for the house physician working in a regional neurological unit. It presupposes a working knowledge of neurological anatomy and physiology and is not meant to supplant the standard reference text-books. It gives a brief account of some facets of neurological examination but this is not intended as a comprehensive description. This guide covers common conditions but inevitably some rarities appear. It is aimed at helping junior doctors to manage the common neurological conditions which lead to emergency admissions and also those neurological problems requiring more elective investigation.

I am indebted to my many colleagues at the Brook and other hospitals for their advice on many topics; also for their referral of patients. I am especially grateful to Dr C. Penney, neuroradiologist at the Brook Hospital, for his help and provision of the X-ray and CT scan pictures. I am also grateful to the photographic department.

I should like to thank Professor Sir John Walton and the Oxford University Press for giving me permission to use Figures 2a and b, and Table IIIa and b, from *Brain's Diseases of the Nervous System*, and to Update Publications for allowing the use of Tables VI, IX and X which are amended from articles originally published by them on 'Strokes' and 'Epilepsy'.

I should also like to acknowledge the great help given by William Heinemann Medical Books in the preparation of the book for publication.

CONTENTS

1. **HISTORY TAKING**
   Preparation of notes, interviews with relatives, consent for investigations and risks, communications, referrals, disturbed patients. 1

2. **NEUROLOGICAL EXAMINATION**
   Higher functions and psychometric assessment, dysphasia, special senses, cranial nerves, motor function, sensation, autonomic function. 3

3. **INVESTIGATIONS**
   Blood tests. Pituitary function and endocrine tests. Cerebrospinal fluid. Electrophysiological tests—EEG, ECG, EMG, evoked potentials. Special eye and ENT tests. 20

4. **RADIOLOGICAL INVESTIGATIONS**
   X-rays — skull, spine, chest. Scans — isotope, RIHSA, CT brain scans. Angiography. Pneumo-encephalography. Myelography. Ventriculography. 26

5. **THE UNCONSCIOUS PATIENT**
   Assessment and examination. Causes of coma and their investigation. Management. 30

6. **THE RESPIRATORY OR INTENSIVE CARE UNIT**
   Respiratory failure, bulbar paralysis, assessment and management. Acute polyneuritis, tetanus, poliomyelitis, myasthenia gravis, status epilepticus. 36

7. **INFECTIONS**
   Meningitis — bacterial, viral, tuberculous — investigations and treatment. Vascular complications. Cerebral abscess. Encephalitis. Herpes zoster. Syphilis. 44

8. **CEREBROVASCULAR DISEASE**
   Acute strokes — embolic, haemorrhagic, thrombotic — investigations, treatment. Cerebral oedema. Sub-arachnoid haemorrhage. Transient ischaemic attacks, management. Hypertensive encephalopathy. Stroke prevention. 54

9. EPILEPSY
Classification, causation, investigation, treatment. Anticonvulsant blood levels. Transient loss of consciousness — causes and investigations. 62

10. HEADACHE
Acute (vascular) migraine, elevated intracranial pressure, cranial arteritis, subdural haematoma. Low pressure headache. Migrainous and trigeminal neuralgia. Chronic headache. Investigations. 69

11. GIDDINESS
Acute paroxysmal attacks, peripheral and central causes. Chronic unsteadiness. Sensory ataxia. Investigations. 73

12. TUMOURS
Elevated intracranial pressure and pressure cones. Focal symptoms and signs, hydrocephalus and endocrine disturbances. Cerebral tumours — in children, in adults — investigations. Treatment of raised intracranial pressure. Features of spinal cord compression, investigations. 76

PLATES 1–16 *between pages* 86 *and* 87

13. SPINAL DEGENERATIVE DISEASE
Cervical and lumbar root involvement, prolapsed intervertebral discs, management. Syringomyelia. 89

14. DEMYELINATING DISEASE
Multiple sclerosis — symptoms, signs, optic neuritis, investigations, management. Acute visual loss. 93

15. DEGENERATIVE DISEASE
Dementia — investigations. Causes — Alzheimer's disease, Huntington's chorea, Jakob-Creutzfeldt's disease, subacute sclerosing panencephalitis, communicating hydrocephalus, multi-infarct dementia. Motor neurone disease. Heredo-familial degenerative disorders — Friedreich's ataxia, peroneal muscular atrophy. 98

16. BASAL GANGLIA DISEASE
    Parkinson's disease, therapy, Involuntary movement disorders. — 104

17. PERIPHERAL NEUROPATHY
    Clinical picture, causation–pressure palsies, B_{12}, B_1 deficiencies. diabetes mellitus, porphyria. Investigations and management. — 108

18. MUSCLE DISEASE AND MYASTHENIA GRAVIS
    Clinical picture, investigations. Dystrophies, myotonia. Polymyositis, polymyalgia rheumatica. Endocrine causes. Myasthenia gravis, diagnosis, management. — 114

19. NEUROLOGICAL MANIFESTATIONS OF SOME MEDICAL DISORDERS
    Deficiencies — thiamine, Wernicke-Korsakoff syndrome, folate. Metabolic — hepatic and renal failure, alcoholism. Endocrine disturbances. Calcium disturbances. Electrolyte disturbances. Connective tissue disorders — rheumatoid arthritis, systemic lupus erythematosus, polyarteritis nodosa. Wegener's granuloma. Sarcoidosis. Neurological syndromes associated with non-metastatic malignancy. — 122

20. HEAD INJURIES
    Acute — assessment, neurosurgical referral. Acute haematoma formation — extra-dural, subdural and intracerebral. Sequelae — epilepsy, CSF leaks. Medico-legal implications. Post-concussive syndrome. — 129

    NORMAL VALUES — 135

    REFERENCES — 138

    INDEX OF PROPRIETARY NAMES — 139

    INDEX — 141

1. HISTORY TAKING

An accurate history is of major importance in making a neurological diagnosis. In most instances, abnormal signs found on examination are those suggested by the history. In many conditions details must be obtained from relatives. This is particularly important in the very young and the elderly. Patients suspected of a presenile dementia with changes of behaviour, memory and personality may give no account of these difficulties which are only too apparent to their relatives. In patients where there is a history of sudden transient loss of consciousness, the account of an observer is probably the most important feature: most types of epileptic fit can be diagnosed from the account of a witness.

Details of *family history* may also be relevant. In many relatively rare neurological disorders, e.g. muscular dystrophies, the family history may help establish the diagnosis. It may be necessary to get accurate details from other hospitals about illness in relatives.

The other parts of the history are also important. Details of past medical history may include accounts of vascular disease, a primary neoplasm, trauma or surgical procedures which may link with patients' current symptoms and signs. With the increasing recognition of the side-effects of drugs, all details of present medication and any past allergies should be recorded. Details of patients' smoking habits and alcohol ingestion should also be entered. If chronic alcoholism is suspected, it is important to question relatives.

Accounts of patients' present symptoms should include their duration, mode of onset, frequency and any aggravating or alleviating factors. Often in more chronic neurological disturbances there may be intermittent or progressive symptoms.

A *social history* is important. Many patients with neurological disease may be left with significant physical, psychological or intellectual deficits which may have to be managed by their family. Patients' occupations may determine the cause of some upsets.

Many hospitals have a set form for entering details of a history and examination. This may prevent omissions but well set out notes in legible writing which contain all the relevant information make the tasks of summary making or referral letters easy. Furthermore if notes have to be produced for medico-legal purposes, inaccuracies, omissions and foolish comments may reflect on the doctor who wrote them.

Information and Risks

Many neurological investigations are invasive procedures. Some are relatively distressing and uncomfortable, others need to be carried out under general anaesthesia. Some have an actual risk of making patients worse. It is important to explain the details of specialised investigations to patients and their relatives, and in the more major neuroradiological procedures and those where surgery is involved, it is necessary to have patients' informed consent. This is usually given by signature on a form. In the very young or in those where their medical or mental state may prevent understanding or the ability to give such consent, then this must be obtained from relatives.

Where the risks and side-effects of a major investigation are well known, e.g. angiography, myelography, some account of these should also be given. Indeed medico-legal problems have arisen when such information has been omitted, and a complication followed. However patients vary in their understanding, fears and reactions to illness and so information may need modification in some instances.

Investigations performed under general anaesthesia also need consent. Furthermore it is important that the junior doctor discuss with his anaesthetic colleagues the fitness of patients for any anaesthetic and alert them to any special risks that patients' neurological conditions might produce, e.g. certain neuromuscular disorders may cause respiratory muscle weakness or abnormal responses to certain relaxant drugs.

Referrals

In neurological units patients may be referred for opinions from consultants in other specialities or for surgery. It is usually the junior doctor's role to arrange such consultations. It is important that the consultant requested is made aware of the question he is being asked and also to give some indication of the urgency of this request. Junior doctors can learn from a visiting specialist's examination and if possible should be present.

Communications

Good communications are essential throughout the investigation, treatment and care of patients in hospital. They involve not only communication with patients and their relatives, but also with other members of staff who may be involved. At the time of discharge or death, patients' general practitioners (and referring consultants) should be informed without delay.

In particular it is the junior doctor's task to assess how ill patients are and to advise the nursing staff about their supervision and care. If they need frequent neurological observations, the frequency should be indicated and also what changes necessitate summoning medical help.

It is wise to visit the patients in your care daily with one of the nursing staff so any changes in patients' conditions can be assessed and any modifications in treatment or nursing discussed. Patients who have undergone any major investigation, e.g. angiography or myelography, should be visited after such a procedure to assess any possible deterioration.

Good communications with other departments and their staff greatly aid the doctor when he seeks their help in a true emergency situation.

Disturbed Patients

In some instances patients under investigation on the ward may prove difficult to manage. Confusional states or alterations in behaviour or personality may pose problems for the staff and other patients.

Various measures may be necessary to overcome such difficulties but it is always important to check there is no physical cause for the upset, e.g. urinary retention. If this is not so, appropriate sedation may allow patients to settle. Rarely patients may be so disturbed that they are dangerous to others or themselves. Here it may be necessary to consider their transfer to a psychiatric unit. Usually it is possible to obtain an acute psychiatric opinion rather than the use of a Section. In an emergency patients can be detained for 72 hours under Section 29 of the Mental Health Act. Such a Section can be made by any registered medical practitioner together with a mental welfare officer.

2. NEUROLOGICAL EXAMINATION

During the history taking, a fair assessment of a patient's conscious level, mental abilities, speech and hearing will usually have been obtained. If there is any clouding of consciousness it is important to have some way of recording this, particularly to see if this is changing. It is suggested that observations based on the Glasgow Coma Scale are used (Teasdale and Jennett, 1974) in

Table I
Coma Scale

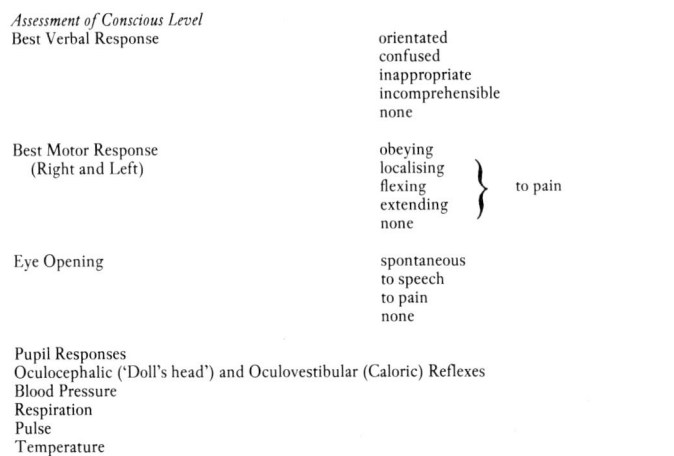

After Teasdale and Jennett (1974)

which the best verbal and motor responses, as well as eye opening are charted (Table I). To these can be added pupillary light reactions, eye movement responses to doll's head manoeuvres (oculo-cephalic reflexes), and records of respiratory rate and rhythm, heart rate, blood pressure and temperature. In acutely ill patients it is important to have such details for a base line on admission as changes in these signs may indicate life-threatening disturbances requiring urgent investigation and treatment. Further details will be given in the chapter on the unconscious patient.

Higher Mental Functions

Some indication of a patient's memory is given by the history. However, simple tests should include questions to check that the patient is orientated in time, place and person. Some details of current events and personalities together with a few questions about the past give information about memory. Repetition of a name and address (eight words) or a Babcock sentence tests immediate memory and repetition after five minutes checks early recall.

Simple calculations or serial subtractions of seven from one hundred, tests memory and in part scholastic attainment. Useful information may be given by relatives of details in a patient's daily performance, e.g. can they dress, lay a table, do the shopping, write a letter, cook a meal etc. Patients sometimes show perseveration, repetition in their replies or responses.

The ability to read, write, copy and draw can also be tested. These involve other functions and should be taken in the context of the patient's schooling. Adult patients still appear who can neither read nor write.

Dysphasia

This describes a disturbance of speech. This is often mixed, in part receptive with impaired understanding, and in part expressive with impaired production. Dysphasia is produced by a dominant hemisphere lesion (probably two thirds of sinistrals have a dominant left hemisphere). With a left frontal lesion there may be non-fluent dysphasia with broken up, telegrammatic speech. Temporal lobe lesions (dominant) produce fluent dysphasia with circumlocutory speech, often with only a few nouns used. Nominal dysphasia causing naming difficulties is also common in temporal lobe lesions. Dyslexia, difficulty reading, dysgraphia, difficulty writing, and dyscalculia, difficulty calculating, usually arise from left parietal lesions.

Psychometric assessment

More formal psychometric assessment is usually made by a clinical psychologist. This should give information about the current level of intellectual function set against the level expected from 'schooling'. The most commonly used test is the Wechsler Adult Intelligence Scale (WAIS). Here a number of sub-tests are used to assess 'verbal' and 'performance' abilities. The scatter of these tests function in different parts of the two hemispheres and brain damage will cause a discrepancy between verbal and performance scores. A number of other tests may be used to assess different functions e.g. Raven's progressive matrices, recognition of famous faces. All these psychometric tests have limitations, perhaps the greatest being the degree of cooperation by the patient.

Special Senses and Cranial Nerves

Cranial Nerve 1: Smell should be tested using a test odour. Many patients appreciate an odour without recognition. Loss may be unilateral. The commonest causes of loss include local nasal disease, head injuries and rarely sub-frontal tumours.

Cranial Nerve 2: The visual acuity should be recorded giving a value for each eye. Snellen test type (at six metres) is used for distance and Jaeger reading cards for near vision. Low vision is recorded as counting fingers (CF), hand movements (HM) or perception of light (PL). If a refractive error is suspected the use of a pin-hole will show improvement in acuity if this is the cause. Ocular causes for impaired vision outnumber optic nerve or visual pathway damage.

The visual fields should be tested using a confrontation technique. The examiner's field is matched against that of the patient for each eye. Major field defects are easily recognised. Small central defects may be missed and here charting on a Bjerrum screen (covers the central $30°$) or the use of a Friedmann analyser (using flashing light patterns at different intensities) will usually show up scotomata. Peripheral field cuts, particularly in chiasmal lesions are best shown by perimetry. A number of machines are available. The Goldmann or Topcon are two which give accurate information and allow the examiner to check continued fixation by the patient during the test. Various patterns of field loss (Fig. 1) may indicate the anatomical site of the lesion in the visual pathways. The use of targets of different sizes and illumination intensities, and of different colour may help to confirm a suspected defect. The blind spot should always be charted.

The optic disc should be examined with an ophthalmoscope, particularly to exclude disc swelling or pallor, the last indicating atrophy. The retina may show abnormalities—haemorrhages, exudates, scars, pigmentary changes and disturbances in the blood vessels e.g. in hypertension or diabetes. Macular lesions are hard to visualise unless the pupil is dilated. Difficulties in examining fundi may be due to changes in the lens or vitreous, or from high refractive errors: in the last instance examining the eyes with patients wearing their glasses may help. Poor fixation or a small pupil may also cause difficulty.

The pupillary response to light, both direct and consensual should be tested. A blind eye has lost the direct light reaction. If the test light is swung quickly from eye to eye then the pupil should constrict each time. An *afferent pupillary defect* describes a pupil that dilates on one side rather than constricts. This occurs if there is a lesion on the afferent pathway between the cornea and chiasm e.g. in optic neuritis.

Optokinetic nystagmus (OKN) is the physiological nystagmus produced by optic fixation on a moving object e.g. looking out of a window in a moving train. It can be tested by showing a patient a revolving striped drum or a moving tape-measure. Parieto-occipital lesions cause a loss of this nystagmus

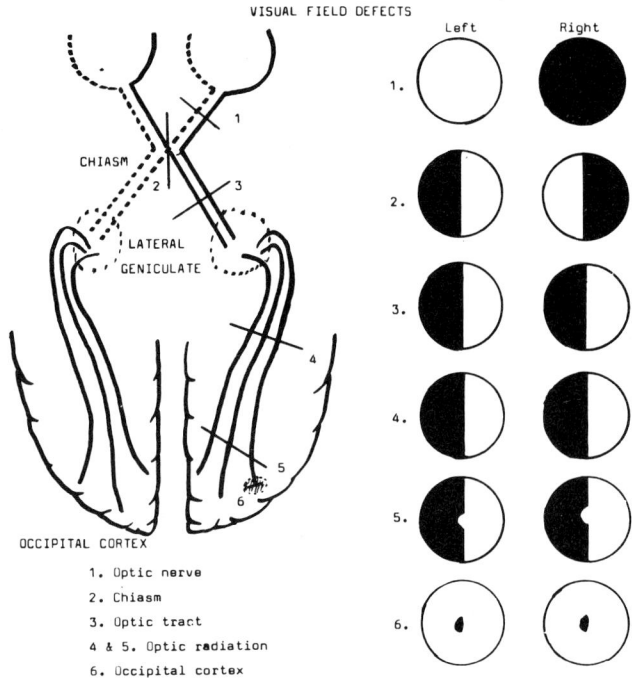

Figure 1

when the 'stripes' are moved towards the side of the lesion. This test may be helpful in showing vision is present in an unco-operative patient or in one feigning blindness.

Cranial Nerves 3, 4 and 6: The oculomotor (3), trochlear (4) and abducens (6) nerves are responsible for eye movements. The lateral rectus muscle (sixth nerve) abducts the eye, and the superior oblique muscle (fourth nerve) is a depressor of the adducted eye, but an intorter of the abducted eye. Thus patients with a trochlear palsy may show a head tilt towards the shoulder opposite to the side of the affected muscle. The other eye muscles are supplied by the third nerve which also supplies the upper lid and pupil. Thus in patients with a complete oculomotor palsy the upper lid droops shut (ptosis), the pupil is dilated and the eyeball abducted: there is loss of adduction, elevation, and depression of the globe.

In addition to the constrictor response of the pupils to light, they also constrict to accommodation and convergence. Paralysis of the sympathetic nervous supply on one side will produce a *Horner's syndrome* with a constricted pupil (miosis), mild ptosis, enophthalmos and impaired sweating on that side of the face. A dilated pupil may be caused by an oculomotor palsy but a *tonic (Adie's) pupil* may present in this way. A tonic pupil commonly occurs in young women and produces a dilated pupil which does not react. In a dark room it reacts very slowly and the iris fibres can be seen to react irregularly under a slit-lamp. Usually there is a slow accommodation response. The diagnosis can be confirmed by demonstrating denervation hypersensitivity in the affected pupil where weak pilocarpine eye drops (0.125%) or methacholine (2.5%) cause constriction. Some patients may have an associated loss of ankle jerks.

Light-near dissociation may be seen in the *Argyll Robertson* pupil. Classically this is a small irregular pupil, unreactive to light but reacting to accommodation. It is usually remembered as a sign of neurosyphilis but may also occur in other mid-brain lesions (in the tectum). *Parinaud's syndrome* describes pupillary light-near dissociation with impaired upgaze and convergence commonly arising from lesions at the level of the superior colliculi e.g. pinealoma.

In examining eye movements, volitional and following (pursuit) movements should be tested. Paralytic lesions of recent onset usually produce diplopia. The two rules for assessing diplopia are (i) to find the direction of gaze which produces the maximal separation of the two images and then (ii) by covering each eye it is possible to show from which eye the false image arises. It is always the most peripheral one. The use of red-green glasses and Hess charting may make analysis easier.

Normally the two eyes move together, conjugate movement. Damage at sites above the level of the oculomotor nuclei may produce conjugate gaze disturbances and these can also occur with damage in the upper brain stem. There are two frontal lobe centres: if one is destroyed, e.g. by a stroke, the eyes will deviate towards the side of the frontal damage from the unopposed action of the intact side. Irritative lesions, as in adversive epileptic fits, arising from one frontal lobe may drive the head and eyes to the opposite side away from where the fit originates. Within the brain stem the median longitudinal fasciculus connects the third and sixth nerve nuclei allowing conjugate horizontal eye movements. Lesions of this pathway, common in multiple sclerosis, produce an *internuclear ophthalmoplegia* with failure of adduction of the eye on the affected side. This is accompanied by coarse nystagmus, 'ataxic', in the abducting eye.

Nystagmus may also be seen during tests of eye movements. Its character, direction, rate and amplitude may all help indicate from where it arises. It implies a break down of the balance of the tone between the opposing ocular muscles and can be produced by disturbances of the retina, eye muscles, vestibular nuclei—their central and peripheral connections (labyrinth, brain stem and cerebellum), by proprioceptive impulses from the neck muscles, and by drugs. Vertical (oscillation in the vertical plane) and rotatory nystagmus usually indicate a central brain stem lesion. Horizontal nystagmus may be of labyrinthine origin, or may arise more centrally or from drugs. *Caloric tests* are based on convection currents induced by temperature change in the semi-circular canals. These are produced by irrigation of the external canals with warm or cold water. This stimulates the brain stem oculo–vestibular connections inducing nystagmus (page 10).

Cranial Nerve 5: The trigeminal nerve is largely sensory: its three divisions supply the face (Fig. 2a, page 18). In addition to testing these areas corneal sensation should be examined. A thin twist of cotton wool is applied to the cornea—the afferent impulse travels through the ophthalmic division which also supplies the inner lining of the nostrils. The efferent impulse travels through the facial nerve to produce a blink. If the last is lost then there may be no blink from the affected side, but there is usually a blink from the unaffected side (the one not tested). In central lesions involving trigeminal sensation there may be loss of pain and temperature only—the area depending on the site of the pontine lesion.

The motor division of the trigeminal nerve supplies the pterygoid, masseter and temporalis muscles. Unilateral paralysis causes deviation of the jaw to the paralysed side and there may be wasting of affected muscles. An exaggerated jaw jerk usually indicates an upper motor neurone lesion above the level of the pons. It is often accompanied by exaggeration of other facial and primitive reflexes. Many of these reflect disturbance in the cortico-bulbar pathways and include the snout, pout, cheek and palmo-mental reflexes. They may be present in normal infants, in the very old and particularly in patients with dementia, and in some with Parkinson's disease or frontal lobe damage. The glabellar tap is a blink produced by tapping the forehead between the eyes; normally this fatigues rapidly but may persist in patients with Parkinson's disease.

Cranial Nerve 7: The facial nerve supplies the facial muscles. It also carries taste from the anterior two thirds of the tongue through the chorda tympani branch which connects the lingual with the facial nerve. Unilateral facial weakness may arise from an upper or lower motor neurone lesion. In the latter the whole of one side of the face is involved with difficulty in eye closure, forehead movement, cheek, lip and mouth movements. In upper motor neurone lesions, weakness is apparent in the lower half of the face on the opposite side. The weakness may be more florid with emotional movements as smiling. Unilateral facial weakness is easy to detect from the asymmetry but bilateral facial weakness, particularly of lower motor neurone type, may be missed as the face may appear symmetrical. Here there will be a bilateral weakness of eye closure and inability to whistle. Primary muscle disease or myasthenia may produce a long, droopy, impassive appearance—myopathic facies.

There are four tastes—salt, sweet, bitter and acid (sour). To test taste in the anterior two thirds, the tongue must be continuously protruded. The test substance is applied to the side of the tongue and after a pause for appreciation, the patient is asked to raise a finger if a taste named by the examiner is recognised. Once the tongue has returned to the mouth, different pathways are stimulated.

Cranial Nerve 8: This has two main divisions, cochlear serving hearing and vestibular supplying the labyrinth. Tests of hearing will detect deafness. If this is present, tests will differentiate conductive (middle ear) from cochlear or perceptive (nerve) deafness. During tests of hearing the side opposite that being tested should be masked e.g. by finger movement in the external meatus. In patients with conductive deafness, sound heard through bone seems louder than that heard through air. Rinne's test uses a vibrating tuning fork (256 cycles) held to the ear and then placed on the mastoid process to compare air with bone conduction. Normally and in nerve deafness air conduction is the better. In Weber's test the vibrating tuning fork is applied to the centre of the forehead. Normally it is heard equally in both ears. In conductive deafness it is loudest in the abnormal ear, in nerve deafness loudest in the normal ear.

Deafness is more accurately assessed by audiometry which is a quantitative measurement of hearing. Various more sophisticated tests of hearing may be undertaken.

Vestibular function is tested in a number of ways. Disturbances of the labyrinth, vestibular nerve or more central connections cause symptoms of vertigo with unsteadiness often associated with nystagmus. *Caloric tests:* water seven degrees above and below body temperature is used for irrigation. This is run into the external canals and if the patient is lying supine with the head flexed to 30° from the horizontal, will stimulate the horizontal semi-circular canals. Normally this produces nystagmus often with vertigo. The mnemonic COWS—Cold Opposite, Warm Same, indicates the direction of the nystagmus (the quick phase) so for example irrigation of the right ear with cold water should produce nystagmus to the left. If nystagmus is absent, a canal paresis is present. This may occur in labyrinthine or vestibular nerve lesions. If the response is reduced in one direction (e.g. warm water in the right and cold water in the left) then this may cause a directional preponderance. This may occur in central lesions e.g. in the vestibular nuclei. Caloric tests should not be performed if the ear drum is perforated.

It is also possible to test for *positional vertigo* and nystagmus. Here the patient sits with the head turned to one side and is told to look up at the examiner's nose. The patient is then laid supine quickly with the neck extended and the head still turned. This stimulates the otolith in the utricle. A lesion at this site causes intense transient vertigo with nystagmus. The nystagmus is usually rotatory in type, appearing after a latent period, and is directed towards the lower ear—the site of the faulty otolith. Repeating the test shows it fatigues and may disappear. Centrally placed lesions in the posterior fossa may cause positional nystagmus and vertigo which has no latent period and does not fatigue. Furthermore the nystagmus may be of varying type, often vertical.

Tests of balance, standing and walking are also very important and are discussed later (page 16).

Cranial Nerves 9 and 10: Speech and swallowing are bulbar functions mediated through the glossopharyngeal and vagus nerves. A patient's voice, ability to cough, swallow and take a drink give good assessment of these functions. Palatal movements can be examined and the 'gag' reflex elicited by applying stimuli to both sides of the back of the throat. There is considerable variation in normal patients to such stimuli. It is possible for the experienced to examine the vocal cords with a laryngeal mirror. A unilateral vagal lesion will cause ipsilateral paralysis of one vocal cord producing a hoarse voice.

Cranial Nerve 11: This supplies the trapezius and sternomastoid. It has a spinal component. The sternomastoid muscles turn the head to the opposite side, so to test the left sternomastoid, the patient should be asked to turn his head to the right pushing against the examiner's hand placed on the right side of the chin. Bilateral weakness may occur in myopathies, myasthenia and motor neurone disease.

Cranial Nerve 12: This supplies the tongue. A lower motor neurone lesion causes wasting of the affected side, with weakness and often visible fasciculation. Attempts at protrusion cause the normal side to push over to the affected side. A bilateral upper motor neurone lesion causes a small contracted tongue which the patient finds hard to move quickly, protrude or produce clear speech. A spastic tongue is often associated with increased facial reflexes and an exaggerated jaw jerk.

Motor Function

Power

Assessment of motor function should include examination of stance and gait. It is useful to look at a patient's ability to perform certain tasks e.g. to climb steps, stand on tip-toe. In many instances the history may suggest patterns of weakness; e.g. proximal leg weakness leads to difficulty getting out of a low chair or bath.

Traditionally weakness is measured on a scale from 0–5 (Medical Research Council, MRC). Total paralysis scores 0, full power 5. Grade 4 indicates normal movement which can be overcome by resistance; grade 3 the muscle can move against gravity but not additional resistance, grade 2 can only move if gravity is eliminated, and grade 1 is a flicker of movement. The difficulty in such an assessment is that there is a very wide range covered by grade 4 and it is often more helpful to record some functional assessment e.g. if the patient can lift a leg from the bed.

To examine muscles, the patient should be fully undressed. This allows muscle wasting to be seen, and also the detection of developmental abnormalities e.g. pes cavus, scoliosis, joint deformities and rarely skin lesions. Wasting may indicate muscle disease, a lesion of the *lower motor neurone* (LMN)—from the anterior horn cell in the spinal cord and distal to it, or less commonly disuse e.g. following immobilisation. The other features of an LMN lesion include the presence of fasciculation, decreased muscle tone and depressed or absent reflexes.

Muscle tone is best assessed by passive movements in a relaxed limb. If relaxation proves difficult, the patient can often be distracted.

Conversely in lesions of the *upper motor neurone* (UMN)—from the cortical motor cells to the anterior horn cell, there may be muscle weakness accompanied by increased tone, clonus, increased tendon reflexes, an extensor plantar response and diminished or absent superficial skin reflexes, e.g. the abdominal reflexes. If the position of the limbs in a patient with a hemiplegia is recalled, the arm and hand are flexed and adducted; the leg is extended with the foot plantar-flexed and inverted. Thus in an UMN lesion the weakness in the arms is more marked in the shoulder abductors, elbow, wrist and finger extensors and the finger abductors. In the leg the hip flexors, hamstrings and the toe and ankle dorsiflexors and evertors are weaker than their antagonists.

Table II
Examination of Limb Muscles

Root	Nerve	Muscle	Action
Arm			
C 5	Circumflex	Deltoid	Shoulder abduction maintained
C 6	Musculo-cutan.	Biceps	Elbow flexion
C 7	Radial	Triceps	Elbow extension
C 8	Median	Flexor dig.	Finger grip
T 1	Ulnar	Dorsal inteross.	Finger abduction
Leg			
L 1	Femoral	Ilio-psoas	Hip flexion
L 2	Obturator	Adductors	Thigh adduction
L 3	Femoral	Quadriceps	Knee extension
L 4	Lat. Popliteal	Tibialis ant.	Ankle dorsiflexion
L 5	Lat. Popliteal	Ext. hallucis	Great toe dorsiflexion
S 1	Med. Popliteal	Gastrocnemius	Ankle plantar flexion
S 2	Med. Popliteal	Flex. digit.	Toe plantar flexion

If weakness is found then other muscles supplied by the same root should be tested using Tables IIIa and b. The myotome overlap is apparent.

Spinal Segment for Tendon Reflexes

Arm		*Leg*	
Biceps	C 5/6	Knee	L 3/4
Triceps	C 7	Ankle	S 1
Finger	C 8		
Supinator	C 5/6		

It is useful to have a quick method of testing muscle power in the limbs. If one muscle supplied predominantly by one nerve root is tested the scheme suggested in Table II may be helpful. If weakness is found then other muscles supplied by that root, or peripheral nerve, should be examined to determine the site of the lesion. There is some overlap so that many muscles have a nerve supply from more than one root. The segmental innervation of the limb muscles are given in Tables IIIa and b.

Weakness may also occur in muscles that fatigue excessively e.g. in myasthenia gravis. In patients where weakness is elaborated often the deficit is global in extent and curious fluctuations can be felt as the muscle contracts. Furthermore agonists and antagonists can be found contracting simultaneously, and discrepancies may appear between performance and formal testing.

Table IIIa *Segmental innervation of Arm Muscles (Courtesy of Professor Sir J. Walton & O.U.P.).*

Region	Muscle	Cervical Segments	Thoracic Segments
		5 — 6 — 7 — 8	1
SHOULDER	Supraspinatus	5–6	
	Teres minor	5–6	
	Deltoid	5–6	
	Infraspinatus	5–6	
	Subscapularis	5–6	
	Teres major	6–7	
ARM	Biceps brachii	5–6	
	Brachialis	5–6	
	Coracobrachialis	6–7	
	Triceps brachii	6–8	
	Anconeus	7–8	
FOREARM	Brachioradialis	5–6	
	Supinator	5–7	
	Extensores carpi radialis	6–7	
	Pronator teres	6–7	
	Flexor carpi radialis	6–7	
	Flexor pollicis longus	6–7	
	Abductor pollicis longus	6–7	
	Extensor pollicis brevis	6–7	
	Extensor pollicis longus	6–7	
	Extensor digitorum communis	6–8	
	Extensor indicis	6–8	
	Extensor carpi ulnaris	6–8	
	Extensor digiti minimi	6–8	
	Flexor digitorum superficialis	7–8	1
	Flexor digitorum profundus	7–8	1
	Pronator quadratus	7–8	1
	Flexor carpi ulnaris	7–8	1
	Palmaris longus	7–8	1
HAND	Abductor pollicis brevis	6–7	
	Flexor pollicis brevis	6–7	
	Opponens pollicis	6–7	
	Flexor digiti minimi brevis	7–8	
	Opponens digiti minimi	7–8	
	Adductor pollicis	8	1
	Palmaris brevis	8	1
	Abductor digiti minimi	8	1
	Lumbricales	8	1
	Interossei	8	1

Table IIIb *Segmental innervation of Leg Muscles*

	T12	L1	L2	L3	L4	L5	S1	S2
HIP	Iliopsoas (T12–L3)				Tensor fasciae latae (L4–S1)			
					Gluteus medius (L4–S1)			
					Gluteus minimus (L4–S1)			
					Quadratus femoris (L4–S1)			
					Gemellus inferior (L4–S1)			
						Gemellus superior (L5–S2)		
						Gluteus maximus (L5–S2)		
						Obturator internus (L5–S2)		
							Piriformis (S1–S2)	
THIGH			Sartorius (L2–L3)					
			Pectineus (L2–L3)					
			Adductor longus (L2–L3)					
			Quadriceps femoris (L2–L4)					
			Gracilis (L2–L4)					
			Adductor brevis (L2–L4)					
				Obturator externus (L3–L4)				
				Adductor magnus (L3–L4)				
				Adductor minimus (L3–L4)				
				Articularis genu (L3–L4)				
LEG					Semitendinosus (L4–S2)			
					Semimembranosus (L4–S2)			
					Biceps femoris (L5–S2)			
				Tibialis anterior (L4–L5)				
				Extensor hallucis longus (L4–S1)				
				Popliteus (L4–S1)				
				Plantaris (L4–S1)				
				Extensor digitorum longus (L4–S1)				
					Soleus (L5–S2)			
					Gastrocnemius (L5–S2)			
				Peroneus longus (L4–S1)				
				Peroneus brevis (L4–S1)				
				Tibialis posterior (L4–S1)				
				Flexor digitorum longus (L4–S2)				
				Flexor hallucis longus (L4–S2)				
FOOT					Extensor hallucis brevis (L4–S1)			
					Extensor digitorum brevis (L4–S1)			
					Flexor digitorum brevis (L5–S1)			
					Abductor hallucis (L5–S1)			
					Flexor hallucis brevis (L5–S1)			
					Lumbricales (L5–S2)			
						Abductor hallucis (S1–S2)		
						Abductor digiti minimi (S1–S2)		
						Flexor digiti minimi brevis (S1–S2)		
						Opponens digiti minimi (S1–S2)		
						Quadratus plantae (S1–S2)		
						Interossei (S1–S2)		

Reflexes

The reflexes are sensory-motor links which may indicate a segmental level of a lesion, or the presence of an UMN or LMN upset. A lesion on the afferent (sensory) side of the arc may produce a depressed or absent reflex. Reflex levels are given in Table II; other tendon reflexes include the jaw, pectoralis and adductor jerks. Superficial skin reflexes include those from the abdomen—upper T 8/9, lower T 11/12, the cremasteric reflexes L 1/2, and the anal reflex S 4/5.

The normal *plantar response (Babinski reflex)* to a firm scratch on the outer border of the sole of the foot is plantar flexion of the great toe. In an UMN lesion the great toe extends (dorsiflexes). Difficulties arise in very cold feet and where there is a brisk withdrawal response of the whole foot and toes. With complete paralysis of the great toe muscles, the response is absent. If the response is difficult to interpret, pricking the dorsum of the great toe with a pin normally causes the toe to move away from the pin. If the response is extensor then the toe may dorsiflex, tending to impale on the pin.

Co-ordination and gait

Fine rapid finger and toe movements allow assessment of a number of facets of motor function. Difficulties will be seen with weakness, extrapyramidal lesions, inco-ordination and gross sensory loss (particularly if position sense is lost). Tests of *co-ordination* should also be performed. Maintaining the arms in an outstretched position, followed by a finger-nose test and fine rapid movements will usually demonstrate any cerebellar limb upset. Tests of stance, gait, hopping and heel-shin test will assess co-ordination in the legs; again many factors influence the responses. *Romberg's sign* demonstrates unsteadiness from proprioceptive loss in the feet. The patient stands with the feet together and then closes the eyes. Mild ataxy (unsteadiness) of stance may be shown by the patient standing tandem (heel to toe) or on one leg. Cerebellar and vestibular lesions may cause patients to fall to one side, or have difficulty walking around a chair.

Much can be detected by a patient's *gait*. The patient with a foot drop lifts the leg high and the affected foot makes a 'slapping' noise as it is placed on the ground. Spastic weakness in a leg or legs may be accompanied by dragging of the affected foot wearing the toe of the shoe. Little short shuffling steps may suggest Parkinson's disease or the 'marche à petits pas' of a patient with widespread cerebrovascular disease.

Sensation

Formal testing of sensation is time consuming and relies on a co-operative patient. Often the history may indicate sensory upset which can be followed e.g. numbness in the extremities may suggest a peripheral neuropathy. Gross areas of sensory loss are easy to demonstrate but in patients with only mild upsets the stimulus intensity may need to be graded to the severity of the symptoms.

Sensations tested include position sense and vibration which travel via the peripheral nerves through the posterior columns in the spinal cord, to the brain stem where they decussate forming the medial fillet. From here they pass into the thalamus and some reach the hemisphere. Some impulses of touch also pass through this pathway. Pain, temperature and some touch sensations pass through peripheral nerves to the cord where the fibres cross and ascend in the spinothalamic tracts. These enter the brain stem passing to the thalamus and sensory cortex.

Two point discrimination and stereognosis follow the same pathways as proprioceptive sensation. Lesions in the parietal cortex cause loss or impairment of these modalities but of course more peripheral sensory lesions will also cause upset of such functions.

The sensory dermatomes and the areas supplied by the major peripheral nerves are given in Fig. 2a, b. There is considerable overlap in the nerve supply of the dermatomes so that if only one nerve root is lost there may be little objective sensory loss. Key points include: C 7 supplies the middle finger in the hand, T 4 is about the level of nipple, T 10 the umbilicus, L 3 lies at the knee, L 5 runs diagonally from the lateral side of the knee to the inner aspect of the foot including the great toe, and S 3, 4 and 5 supply a circular area in the perineum radiating out from the anus (including the scrotum in the male). If sensory loss is found, it is worth charting this: it aids in anatomically placing the lesion and in following progress.

Autonomic Function

Autonomic upset usually causes disturbance in bowel, bladder and sexual functions. The rectum is a reservoir so defects of innervation produce constipation. However if the patient develops diarrhoea then faecal soiling may occur. In normal subjects pricking or scratching the anal skin causes contraction of the external sphincter, the anal reflex. A patulous anus suggests gross denervation from sacral segmental loss. Various neurogenic bladder upsets may occur often leading to urgency and frequency of micturition, later

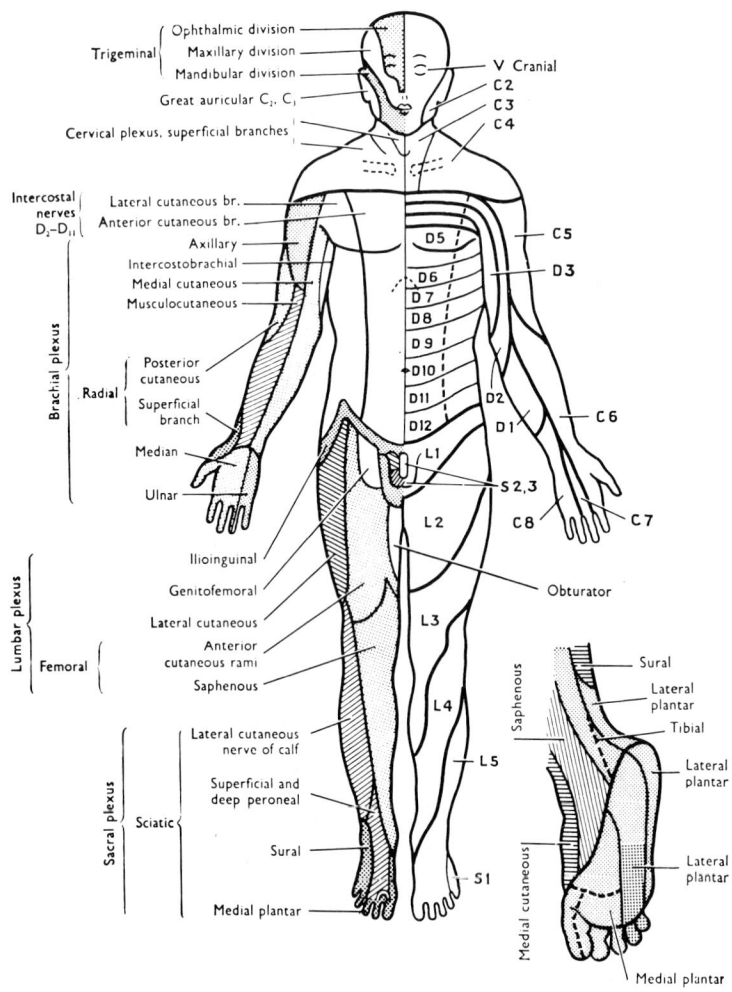

ANTERIOR ASPECT

Figure 2a: *Sensory areas supplied by spinal segments and peripheral nerves. (Courtesy of Professor Sir J. Walton & O.U.P.).*

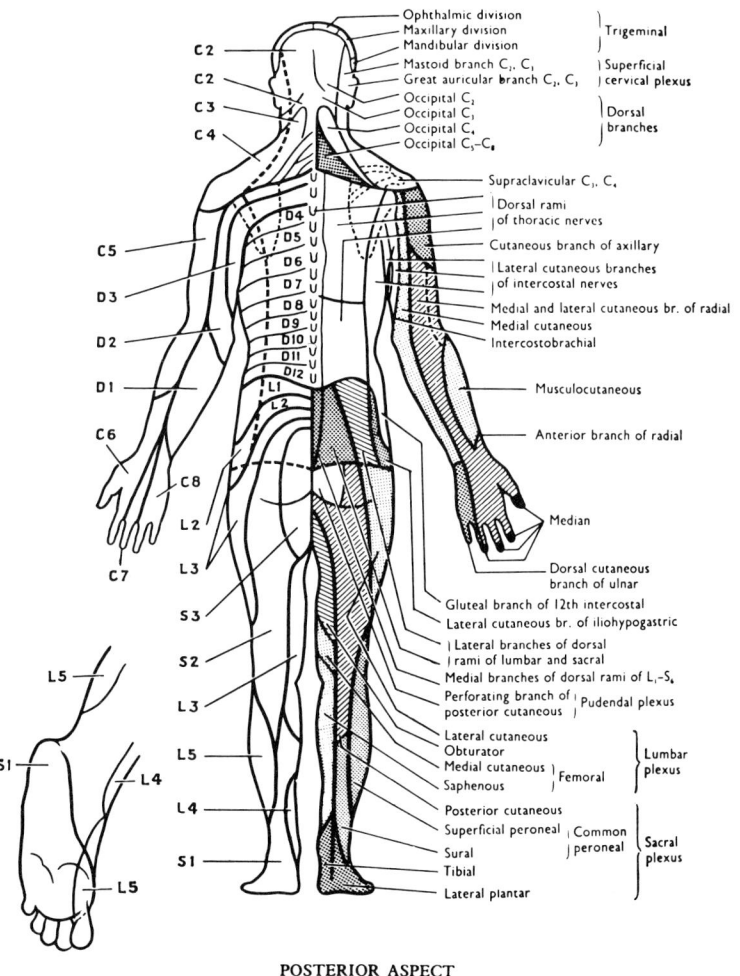

Figure 2b: *Sensory areas supplied by spinal segments and peripheral nerves.*

hesitancy and retention with overflow. An LMN lesion of the bladder (or loss of afferent input) causes a large flaccid bladder with dribbling incontinence. Although many causes of impotence are psychogenic, spinal cord lesions and cauda equina disturbances may produce impotence as an early symptom.

Sweating and the pupillary responses also have an autonomic supply. In severe disturbances sweating is lost and there may be complaints of blurred vision. In patients suspected of having an autonomic neuropathy, the blood pressure standing and lying should be taken for there may be a marked postural drop. More sophisticated chemical tests may also be necessary.

A *full general examination* should always be undertaken.

Examination of *small children* leads to difficulties for the inexperienced. Observations from parents are very helpful and watching a child at play or other daily tasks yields much information. There are many useful assessment tables giving the expected age for children to achieve certain milestones. They also show the height, weight and skull circumference for that age e.g. *Paediatric Vade-Mecum*, edited by Wood (1974).

In children with neurological upset it is very important to discover if this is static or progressive.

3. INVESTIGATIONS

Appropriate investigations should be chosen based on the history and examination. Some hospitals rely on a screening profile for a number of biochemical tests: this method has its advocates but important individual tests should not be omitted.

Most hospitals provide medical staff with details of requirements for certain blood tests and lists of normal values. It is wise to know these so that samples can be correctly taken. A list of normal values is given (pages 135–137) but individual laboratories may show some variation.

Most neurological patients should have blood taken for (1) a full blood count (FBC) and sedimentation rate (ESR), (2) a screening serological test (WR +) to exclude syphilis (page 52), and (3) estimation of glucose, urea and electrolytes. In patients with a depressed conscious level of unknown cause, blood should also be taken for liver function tests and a sample kept for drug analysis.

Endocrine Studies

In patients suspected of endocrine disorders appropriate tests can be made from blood samples. Diabetes mellitus can be excluded by a fasting and two hour post-prandial blood glucose level; a full glucose tolerance test may sometimes be necessary.

Pituitary function involves different tests to assess the drive to various distant endocrine glands. Secreting tumours will give increased hormone levels e.g. prolactin. When *hypopituitarism* is suspected a *'triple bolus test'* will show if this is present. The test is based on producing hypoglycaemia to act as a stress to stimulate the gland. Patients with florid hypopituitarism do not need this. The test should not be performed in patients with ischaemic heart disease or epilepsy. Patients being tested should remain under constant supervision so that dangerous hypoglycaemia is not produced. If it is, intravenous (IV) glucose can be used to correct it.

An indwelling needle is placed in a large vein in a fasting patient. Blood is taken for base line values of glucose, thyroxine, growth hormone (GH), cortisol, prolactin, adrenocorticotrophic hormone (ACTH), thyroid stimulating hormone (TSH), follicle stimulating hormone (FSH) and luteinising hormone (LH). At the start intravenous injections are given serially of:

1. soluble insulin $0.1 - 0.15$ units/kg body weight. This should produce hypoglycaemia with symptoms and a blood glucose less than 2.2 mmol/l. If not the stimulus is inadequate.

2. 200 µg thyrotrophin-releasing hormone (TRH), and

3. 100 µg FSH/LH-releasing hormone.

Blood samples are taken at;

20 minutes for TSH, prolactin, FSH & LH,

30 minutes for glucose, GH, cortisol, ACTH, prolactin,

60 minutes for glucose, GH, cortisol, ACTH, prolactin, TSH, FSH & LH,

90 minutes for glucose, GH, cortisol, ACTH, prolactin,

120 and 180 minutes for glucose, GH, and cortisol.

In normal patients the blood glucose falls and then rises. Cortisol values with an excess of 450 nmol/l, and GH values of greater than 20 mu/l should be found. Normally the prolactin value rises $\times 3$ in men and $\times 6$ in women. With TRH normally the TSH values should lie between 5–20 mu/l at 20 minutes and 2–18 mu/l at 60 minutes. Values for FSH and LH vary with sex and age: post menopausal women have high basal values. In males basal values of FSH are 1–6 IU/l and LH 2–9 IU/l. After FSH/LH releasing hormone there is usually a peak value arising after 20–30 minutes. LH should increase by at least five times the basal value and FSH by an increment of > 1.5.

Thyroid function can be screened by a thyroxine level (T4) and a tri-iodothyronine level (T3). Estimates of TSH may be helpful in detecting hypothyroidism and radio-iodine uptake studies may also be useful.

Adrenal function can be measured by estimating plasma cortisol levels. Normally there is a diurnal rhythm, values being highest in the early morning and lowest at midnight. Urinary estimations of 17 hydroxycorticosteroids and oxogenic steroids may also be useful particularly if Cushing's disease is suspected. ACTH levels will differentiate those due to a secreting pituitary lesion. Electrolyte disturbances also occur.

Diabetes insipidus was formerly diagnosed on the results of fluid balance studies, followed by a water deprivation test. Oral fluids are restricted for eight hours and in normal patients the urine will concentrate as the plasma solute concentration rises. Now osmolality measurements are made on samples of plasma and urine in the first hour, and in the hours between three and four, six and seven, and seven and eight. In normal patients the urine osmolality will rise to 600 mosm/kg or more but the plasma osmolality will not rise above 300 mosm/kg. In diabetes insipidus the plasma value will rise above 300 while the urine remains dilute at less than 270 mosm/kg.

Certain other tests may prove valuable. Patients suspected of alcoholic induced liver damage should have routine liver function tests including the aspartate aminotransferase (AST) and gamma glutamyltranspeptidase (γGT). Suspicions of B_1 deficiency can be confirmed by a red cell transketolase which has largely replaced the pyruvate tolerance test.

Primary muscle disease may produce an elevated creatine phosphokinase (CK) level. Mild increases may be helpful in carrier detection in certain dystrophies. Massive muscle or tissue damage will cause a rise in CK.

Rare metabolic disorders may be detected by specific tests e.g. phytanic acid in the blood in Refsum's disease, or the presence of porphyrins in the urine in porphyria.

Cerebrospinal Fluid (CSF)

CSF examination is essential in patients suspected of meningitis or a subarachnoid haemorrhage (SAH). It carries a real risk in patients with raised intracranial pressure (ICP) as it may produce a pressure cone. Furthermore it is contra-indicated in patients suspected of having a cerebral tumour or abscess.

The spinal cord usually ends in adults at the lowest border of the first lumbar vertebra so fluid can be safely obtained from the subarachnoid space below this level. A line joining the tops of the iliac crests crosses the L 3/4 interspace and this is often the best position to insert the needle. It is worth spending time correctly positioning patients lying on their side, fully flexed with the spine in a horizontal line. The procedure should be performed with full aseptic precautions; local skin sepsis is a contra-indication. Local anaesthetic should be used in the skin and immediate tissues and then a sharp disposable lumbar puncture needle with stilette inserted and advanced slowly through the space between the two spinous processes. Usually a slight 'give' is felt as the needle penetrates the dura. Normal CSF is crystal clear. The pressure should be measured with a manometer.

In patients suspected of a spinal compressive lesion myelography is usually performed. However in such patients intermittent compression of the jugular veins in the neck (Queckenstedt's test) can be used to test if there is a free rise and fall in the venous pressure which is transmitted to the CSF pressure providing there is no spinal block.

Three samples of CSF are taken, one being placed in a fluoride tube for glucose estimation. Normal values are given on p. 136. A sample of blood for glucose estimation should also be taken at the same time. An infected fluid often appears milky. If there has been a traumatic tap causing the appearance of blood stained fluid, this may run clear in successive specimens. In all such instances the laboratory should be asked to centrifuge the specimens and check that the supernatant is clear. In fresh specimens a xanthochromic supernatant suggests a recent haemorrhage.

Recent studies have shown the CSF lactate is elevated (> 3.3 mmol/l) in bacterial and tuberculous meningitis, whereas in normal patients and those with a viral meningitis the value is low (usually < 2.8 mmol/l). The levels fall with antibiotic treatment and are only reliable when there is a CSF pleocytosis of > 10 cells/mm^3.

In tuberculous meningitis (TBM) the blood-brain barrier becomes more permeable and this is used as the basis for a diagnostic test measuring the ratio of concentrations of bromide in blood and CSF. In normal patients the blood bromide concentration is about three times that in the CSF. Bromide can be given orally (1.0 g t.i.d for three days) or IV (8.0 g in 30 ml) and on the following day, a sample of blood and CSF are taken for bromide estimation. Values less than 1.6 suggest TBM. An isotopic method is also available.

Cisternal puncture should only be performed by the very experienced operator. It is not a procedure for the houseman in training unless under strict supervision for if the needle is advanced too far it may enter the medulla with fatal results.

Electrophysiological Studies

These are largely non-invasive and may add useful information but they require careful selection and interpretation.

The Electroencephalogram (EEG): records wave forms produced by electrical activity in the surface neurones of the brain recorded through surface scalp electrodes with much amplification. Numerous artefacts need recognition Basically four rhythms are described; alpha 8–12, beta greater than 12, theta 4–7, and delta less than three c.p.s. (Hz). Various physiological activities alter these rhythms such as sleep, or overbreathing. Diffuse disturbances may occur with metabolic or vascular upsets producing slower rhythms. With recovery these will improve. Structural focal lesions, as tumours or abscesses, may show a local slow wave abnormality.

In the investigation of patients with transient loss of consciousness the EEG may be helpful if the record shows paroxysmal discharges, or a local spike focus, e.g. in one temporal lobe. However EEG changes are not pathognomonic of epilepsy and some 10–15% of the 'normal' population have 'abnormal' records. Furthermore a 'normal' EEG does not exclude a diagnosis of epilepsy. In a few rare conditions the EEG may largely make the diagnosis, e.g. herpes simplex encephalitis, or Jakob-Creutzfeldt disease.

The Electrocardiogram (ECG): helps detect cardiac arrhythmias, abnormalities of conduction or cardiac damage. Rare neuromuscular disorders, particularly some dystrophies and spino-cerebellar degenerations, may be accompanied by ECG changes. In patients with acute cerebral haemorrhage or SAH, ST depression and T wave inversion may appear. In patients with recent strokes or transient ischaemic attacks (TIAs), an ECG may show a cardiac source for emboli. In some patients with transient disorders as dizziness or faint feelings, paroxysmal changes of cardiac rate or rhythm may be responsible, which may only be detected by the use of a continuous ECG record. Ambulatory cardiac monitoring is now possible using a portable machine, but it is important for patients to put a signal on the tape at the time when they have symptoms for asymptomatic changes may occur.

The Electromyogram (EMG): is a diagnostic extension of clinical examination. It is possible to stimulate certain peripheral nerves and record signals from them. Conduction velocities and amplitudes of action potentials can be measured. These give an accurate means of assessing whether conduction in large fast-conducting peripheral nerve fibres is normal. Nerves are made up of many thousands of fibres and the amplitude of the compound action potential is a measure of the contribution of these fibres, if the nerve is stimulated supramaximally. Diminution in amplitude may indicate fall-out of conducting fibres, as may occur in axonal degeneration. Loss or thinning of the myelin sheath in fibres may cause conduction block or marked slowing of conduction velocity.

Muscle sampling with a concentric needle electrode gives information about the muscle and its innervation. Specific patterns are seen with voluntary muscle contraction which differ when a muscle is partially or severely denervated. The presence of fibrillation usually indicates denervation, although rarely may occur in polymyositis. Primary muscle disease yields a distinct pattern with short duration low amplitude polyphasic potentials.

EMG studies may show the presence of a subclinical neuropathy and are particularly helpful in demonstrating the site of local nerve 'entrapment' lesions, e.g. in the carpal tunnel.

Evoked Potentials: these can be measured with the aid of sophisticated electrical recording equipment, usually through surface electrodes from various areas of the brain and spinal cord, after an appropriate peripheral stimulus. Although many methods are still experimental, visual and to a lesser extent auditory and spinal evoked potentials have proved their value. For visual stimulation an alternating checkerboard pattern is used and the visual evoked responses (VERs) recorded from the occipital cortex. Conduction delay in the visual pathways, as may occur in demyelination in optic neuritis, is clearly shown. This test may prove positive in patients who have no clear clinical history of visual upset but who have had a subclinical episode of optic neuritis. However conduction delay is not pathognomonic for optic neuritis.

Other Tests

In the eye clinic a number of other tests may also be performed. Intraocular pressure may be measured to exclude glaucoma. Serial retinal photography may be combined with an IV injection of the dye, fluorescein. This gives details of the retinal vasculature, and will also show delayed and persistent leakage of the dye from the optic disc if that is swollen. This is very useful if there is doubt as to whether the optic disc is swollen from raised pressure or if there is local pathology, as a buried drusen.

In ENT departments routine audiometry and caloric tests are often combined with more detailed tests of hearing to show the anatomical site for any deafness. Electronystagmography (ENG) allows the recording of eye movements electrically and will show up patterns of nystagmus which may alter significantly when fixation is lost, as in the dark. Such patterns may help to differentiate peripheral from central vestibular lesions. About two thirds of patients with peripheral lesions show spontaneous nystagmus which enhances with eye closure, or in the dark. In others such measures provoke nystagmus. In central lesions spontaneous nystagmus may be in different directions, even vertical, and usually disappears with eye closure, or in the dark. However a few patients with vestibular disturbance show no nystagmus under any conditions.

Rotational tests may also be used.

4. RADIOLOGICAL INVESTIGATIONS

Good quality X-rays are important. It is better to obtain such films in acutely ill patients at a time when they can best co-operate. Restless, confused patients provide poor quality films which may prove worthless.

Skull X-rays should include lateral, PA, Towne's and basal views.

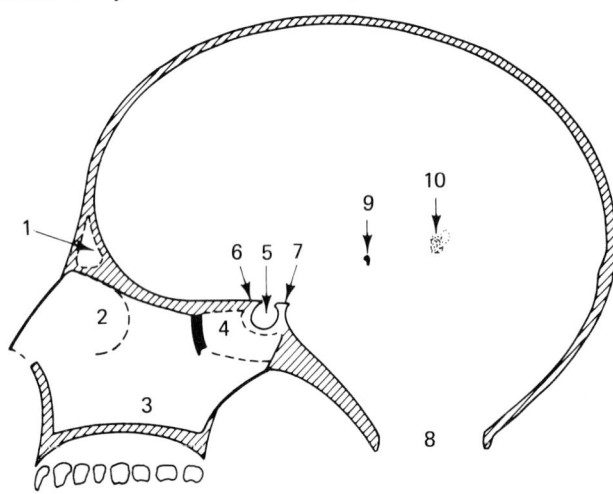

Important features in a lateral skull X-ray

1	Frontal sinus	6	Anterior clinoids
2	Orbit	7	Dorsum sellae
3	Hard palate	8	Foramen magnum
4	Sphenoid sinus	9	Pineal (if calcified)
5	Pituitary fossa	10	Choroid plexus (if calcified)

Figure 3

Raised ICP may be shown by loss of the lamina dura in the dorsum sellae followed by erosion. In children, prior to fusion of the skull sutures, raised ICP may cause splaying of the sutures or delay in their fusion. The so-called 'beaten pewter' appearance of the skull may be present with raised ICP but this is not a reliable sign.

An intrasellar pituitary tumour may balloon the fossa, sometimes asymmetrically. A sella measuring more than 12 mm deep and 16 mm long (on the lateral film) is usually abnormal (Plate 1). Local tumours above the sella or even a dilated third ventricle, may erode the top of the dorsum sellae.

In nearly 50% of adults the pineal gland is calcified. Unilateral supratentorial masses may cause displacement ($>$ 3 mm) to one side and such shifts are significant on symmetrical films. Bilateral subdural haematomata and some other masses may cause downward displacement of the pineal. Choroid plexus calcification is less common and when asymmetrical may cause problems. Calcification may appear in arteriosclerotic arteries, particularly in the elderly, and in some patients in the falx. Pathological calcification may occur in tumours (Plates 2a, b), commonly in slow growing gliomas, and in some meningiomata. The latter may also show hyperostosis at the site of attachment to the skull. Lytic areas in the skull may arise from metastatic deposits but more commonly low density areas in the vault may be produced by venous lakes.

Asymmetry in size of the various foramina in the skull may indicate nerves thickened by masses, e.g. a difference of more than two mm in the diameter of the internal auditory canals in the petrous bones suggests the presence of an acoustic neuroma on the expanded side.

Chest X-rays should always be taken in all adult neurological patients. They may show unexpected pathology such as multiple metastatic shadows or hilar gland enlargement. Apical shadows may be missed and are of great relevance in patients with Horner's syndrome or brachial symptoms. The cardiac size and contour may suggest certain patterns of heart disease.

Spinal X-rays require good quality films particularly in the fat and elderly. The appropriate site of a suspected spinal lesion should always be clearly indicated to the radiologist and sometimes discussion may help in obtaining appropriate special views or tomograms. All too often films of the lumbar spine are requested in patients with a spastic weakness of the legs i.e. below the level of the end of the spinal cord.

Normally the bony confines of the spinal canal can be shown and so any narrowing, widening or angulation can be seen. Developmental defects may be shown. Oblique views of the intervertebral (exit) foramina may show widening or encroachment by osteophytic spurs. Prolapsed discs may cause narrowing of a disc space and less often calcification. Figures are available for the lateral diameter of the spinal canal; in the cervical region values of 10–11 mm suggest a possible myelopathy from compression within a narrow canal.

Other X-ray investigations may be indicated by patients' symptoms and signs, e.g. an intravenous pyelogram or micturating cine cystometrogram may be helpful in the assessment of patients with possible neurogenic bladder disturbance.

Scanning

Isotope (radionucleide) scans rely on the differential uptake by certain tissues of various isotopes. By scanning the area under test with a gamma camera it is possible to show such uptake and in particular areas of abnormality. In the brain technetium is the isotope most commonly used. It will show up most meningiomata, metastases, abscesses and a proportion of gliomas. Lesions in the posterior fossa and para-pituitary areas are poorly demarcated and certain tumours at these sites may be missed. Cerebrovascular lesions give a variable yield. With appropriate timing of the scan (after 5 – 7 days from the ictus) many supratentorial infarcts may be shown. If the scan is repeated some six weeks later many such lesions have disappeared.

Other types of isotope scan, such as liver or bone scans, may be indicated.

Radio-iodinated Human Serum Albumin (RIHSA) scans use isotopic labelled albumin which is injected by lumbar puncture into the CSF. The distribution and absorption of the isotope is then determined by scanning the head at certain time intervals. In patients with obstruction of the CSF pathways or failure of absorption, abnormal patterns may be detected. It can also be used to detect the patency of 'shunts' and to delineate CSF fistulae.

Computerised tomography (CT) is now used in brain scanning and is the investigation of choice for patients suspected of brain disease. Here a collimated X-ray beam scans 'slices' of brain at different levels using a tomographic method. The differential absorption of X-rays by the tissue scanned is processed through a computer which usually produces a visual display. This allows delineation of brain tissue and the ventricular cavities so that any displacements or enlargements are well shown. Abnormal absorption may occur in areas of damage whether from trauma, infection (abscesses), tumours, infarcts, or haemorrhages. With the use of an intravenous injection of iodine-containing contrast medium it is possible to enhance certain areas of abnormal density, particularly if these are very vascular. The radiation dose is low, the procedure quick and well tolerated so that it can be done as an outpatient test. In very young children, or restless or confused patients who cannot lie still a general anaesthetic may be necessary.

CT scans are most useful in tumour diagnosis, in the demonstration of atrophic processes, in showing hydrocephalus, in detecting abscesses, haematomata (subdural, extradural and intracranial), and in the management of patients with cerebrovascular diseases (Plates 3–10). Because of limited availability selection of patients is necessary.

Echo-encephalography in the hands of experts may be useful in detecting intracranial supratentorial shifts from the midline. Here an ultrasound probe is used to delineate echoes from various cranial structures. Difficulties may arise in determining the midline echo. This is a helpful test, particularly in patients where there is no visible pineal calcification.

Carotid and Vertebral Angiography involves the intra-arterial injection of contrast media either through a needle or a catheter inserted via a needle. Angiography is still necessary to show intracranial aneurysms, certain vascular malformations (angiomata) and the blood supply of certain tumours. It is also useful in showing disease in extracranial feeding arteries which may be the source of emboli in patients with TIAs (Plates 11 a, b; 12). It is still used to investigate patients suspected of an intracranial mass where CT scanning is not available.

Unfortunately it is an uncomfortable procedure and so is commonly performed under general anaesthetic. It carries a small but definite mortality and morbidity. The risks are highest in older patients with vascular disease and in the hands of unskilled operators.

Pneumo-encephalography (PEG or AEG) involves the injection of air through a lumbar puncture needle which passes into the ventricular system and cisterns around the brain. By moving the patient it is possible to move the air, like a bubble in a spirit level, to outline the ventricles and often the CSF spaces over the surface of the brain.

It is an invasive procedure which is unpleasant usually producing severe headache which may persist for some days. Because of this it may be performed under general anaesthetic and now modern rotating X-ray chairs help in the movement of the 'unconscious' patient. It carries some risk and if there is an intracranial mass may alter the pressure relationships and provoke a pressure cone. It is a very good way of showing cerebral atrophy although now has largely been replaced by the CT scan. It is still of value in showing small mass lesions in the para-pituitary region.

Myelography uses the injection by lumbar puncture of a radio-opaque dye into the subarachnoid space. The dye is used to show up the spinal cord and its roots within the spinal canal. Iodophendylate (Myodil, Pantopaque) is the most commonly used dye. Six to nine ml of this is injected and as it is heavier than CSF it can be moved by gravity. The patient is strapped to a tipping X-ray table and the movement of the dye screened with the patient in the prone and supine position. This allows the dye to run along the whole spinal canal from the lumbo-sacral sac to the foramen magnum. Any obstruction or persistent filling defect in the column can be seen, as can any expansion of the spinal cord (Plates 14–16a).

Iodophendylate (Myodil) in some patients proves somewhat irritant and complaints of back pain radiating to the buttocks and legs may occur afterwards. These may be accompanied by a degree of 'chemical' meningism. Rarely reports of an adhesive arachnoiditis following myelography have been made and because of these many operators try to remove as much dye as possible after the procedure. This involves a further lumbar puncture and dye removal under X-ray control.

More recently water-soluble iodine-containing contrast media have been tried. Initially these were only useful for radiculograms as the dye was too irritant to run over the spinal cord. However, metrizamide (Amipaque) is a water-soluble medium which can be run over the cord and roots without upset. This is now increasingly used, although it disappears within an hour of injection.

Air is sometimes used as a contrast medium in myelography and this may prove very useful in children, also in certain conditions in adults, e.g. in demonstrating a syrinx with tonsillar herniation through the foramen magnum.

Ventriculography involves the injection of air, or sometimes an iodine-containing contrast medium, into the ventricles. This requires surgery to make a burr hole and then a needle is passed through brain tissue into the ventricles. It is most easily performed in patients with enlarged ventricles and will show the presence of an obstructive hydrocephalus, distortion or shifts of the ventricles. It is an invasive procedure and in patients with masses causing elevated pressure or displacements, may precipitate coning. Because of this it is often carried out prior to more definitive surgery.

5. THE UNCONSCIOUS PATIENT

Depression or clouding of consciousness is an important sign. Different degrees may be recognised but definitions vary making assessment difficult.

Comatose patients are unconscious, unresponsive to verbal commands and often to painful stimuli. In some patients primitive responses e.g. limb withdrawal or extension, can be elicited by painful stimuli. An international coma scale has been suggested: the Glasgow scale (Teasdale and Jennett, 1974) which has proved practical and reliable for doctors and nurses. This records eye opening and best verbal and motor responses (Table I, page 4).

Drowsiness resembles normal sleep so patients can be roused by stimulation to wakefulness and will co-operate, but if left alone will fall asleep again. *Stupor* usually indicates unconscious patients who can be roused to resist painful stimuli for short periods, and even produce verbal responses but who do not co-operate. When the stimulation ceases patients again lose consciousness. A *persistent vegetative state* causes absence of any function of the cerebral cortex. Such patients do not speak or respond in any purposeful way, although may show periods of wakefulness, produce grunts and even show primitive reflex limb movements. The '*locked-in*' syndrome describes patients who have sustained motor damage in the pons causing limb paralysis and speech loss. However they can hear, see and understand so communication may be possible using eye blinking or facial movements. *Akinetic mutism* is used to describe patients who lie immobile, making no speech or sound, but who can follow with their eyes. Such patients often appear about to say something or respond.

Confusion suggests patients who are alert but incorrect in their orientation for time, place or even person. Disorientation in time is the most common. *Delirious* patients appear confused and out of touch with their surrounds. They are often restless and show motor overactivity so that they become physically exhausted. Although alcoholic withdrawal is one cause, such toxic confusional states may occur, particularly in the elderly, with acute infections, anoxia or metabolic upsets.

Examination

An immediate record of conscious level should be made and charted. *Respiratory function* should be assessed checking that the airway is clear. Vomit, excess secretions or loose dentures obstructing the mouth should be removed. The pattern of breathing may be disordered: such upsets may follow local lung disease or certain metabolic disturbances. Shallow rapid breathing may occur in shock or hypoglycaemia. Brain damage alters the respiratory pattern in some patients: Cheyne-Stokes respiration describes a waxing and waning pattern where periods of apnoea alternate with overbreathing and may follow bihemisphere damage or metabolic upset such as uraemia. Rapid regular overbreathing, central neurogenic hyperventilation, occurs with high brain stem lesions. Damage lower down in the pons and medulla causes irregular breathing often with apneustic gaps or clusters of irregular breaths.

The *pupillary responses* should be assessed and charted. As discussed, a fixed dilated pupil on one side suggests a third nerve lesion which may be due to a pressure cone. Bilateral fixed and dilated pupils suggest significant brain stem damage which may prove irreversible. Care should be taken to check that no mydriatic eye drops have been used. Damage at certain levels of the brain stem may cause pupillary changes: pontine lesions often produce very small, 'pinpoint' pupils. Mid-brain lesions may cause pupils in the mid-position, often fixed but sometimes showing fluctuations in size. Certain drugs cause pupillary changes: opiates and codeine will produce small pupils: glutethimide poisoning moderately dilated pupils. Severe drug overdoses or anoxia (e.g. after cardiac arrest) may cause fixed dilated pupils.

Eye movements may still occur spontaneously in patients with a depressed conscious level and intact brain stem function. Break down of eye movements may occur with an oculomotor or abducens palsy. Derangements of conjugate gaze usually suggest a local structural lesion. Tonic deviation of the eyes to one side may follow damage to the frontal region (on the ipsilateral side), or a lesion in the pons (where the eyes are turned away from the side of the lesion). Paralysis of upward gaze suggests a compressive lesion at the level of the tectal plate in the mid-brain. In the unconscious patient eye movements can be tested by the 'doll's head' manoeuvre (oculo-cephalic reflex). If the patient's head is held between the examiner's hands which hold the eyes open, rotation from side to side, and flexion and extension should be accompanied by contraversive conjugate deviation of the eyes. Eye movements can also be assessed by the caloric test (oculo-vestibular reflex). In an unconscious patient ice-cold water can be used which is a very potent stimulus. If the patient has intact brain stem function there will either be nystagmus in the direction away from the ear irrigated, or conjugate deviation of the eyes to the irrigated side.

A *full neurological examination* should be performed particularly noting any voluntary or involuntary limb movements, odd postures and any lateralising changes in the tone and reflexes.

In the face, lash and corneal reflexes should be tested and the 'gag' reflex elicited from the throat. In testing the corneal reflex there is often a bilateral blink or upward deviation of the eyes if brain stem function is intact.

In patients with acute lesions involving the corticospinal tract, the affected limbs may initially appear flaccid, with depressed tendon reflexes but extensor plantar response. After a variable time the tone and reflexes increase. Lifting the arms and legs and letting them fall may elicit such differences. In assessing sensation, patients' reactions to painful stimuli may be observed. Grimacing, withdrawal of the limb or even pupillary dilatation may occur if sensation is preserved. Failure of any movement in limbs on one side suggests sensory loss or paralysis. Signs of *decorticate rigidity* may appear when stimulation produces flexion of the arm and extension of the leg—the position of hemiplegic limbs. These signs often follow damage to the corticospinal tract within the hemisphere. Signs of *decerebrate rigidity* are shown by arching of the back, and extension of the arms and legs. Commonly such patients have sustained damage to the mid-brain or lower down the brain stem but severe anoxia, drug intoxication, or metabolic coma which all depress the upper brain stem, may produce such signs.

The optic fundi should be examined for disc swelling, haemorrhages, or any form of retinopathy. The ears should be examined for signs of local infection or bleeding. Blood behind the ear drum may suggest a basal skull fracture.

The circulatory system should be examined and the blood pressure and pulse rate recorded. The peripheral pulses should be checked. General examination should include a search for any signs of a primary neoplasm, lymphadenopathy or the stigmata of liver failure.

The temperature should be recorded and patients tested for signs of meningeal irritation—neck stiffness or the the presence of Kernig's sign. If the meninges are inflamed then it is impossible to extend the knee fully when the leg is flexed to 90° at the hip (Kernig positive). In the very young, the very old and in some critically ill patients with meningitis, signs of meningism may be absent.

The skull should be examined for any signs of injury or past neurosurgical intervention. In infants a bulging anterior fontanelle may indicate elevated ICP.

Causes of Coma (Table IV)

In a general hospital, *self-poisoning* by drugs or alcohol is still the most common cause: careful inquiry from relatives or attendants may give the diagnosis. In coma of *metabolic origin* there are often clues in the past history. Diabetes mellitus is the most common cause. In the insulin-treated diabetic *hypoglycaemic* attacks may occur. These are usually manifest by episodic confusion, irritability, disturbed behaviour and agitation before loss of consciousness. Dysarthria, ataxia, and complaints of blurred or double vision may

Table IV
Causes of Coma

Self Poisoning	{ Drugs Alcohol	
Metabolic	Diabetes mellitus	{ hypoglycaemic ketotic hyperosmolar
	Uraemia	
	Hepatic Failure	
	Thiamine deficiency (Wernicke)	
Endocrine	Myxoedema	
	Pituitary apoplexy	
Anoxia	Cardiac causes	{ arrest post-surgery
	Respiratory causes	{ lung disease 'Gas' poisoning
Neurological Causes		
Trauma	Head injuries	{ acute injury compressive haematoma
Infection	Meningitis	
	Encephalitis	
	Abscess	
Tumours	Primary	
	Metastatic	
Cerebrovascular Disease	Thrombo-embolic infarction	
	Haemorrhage	{ Primary Sub-arachnoid (SAH)
Epilepsy		

occur raising the possibility that patients are drunk. Occasionally there may be focal neurological signs. A low blood glucose releases adrenaline which produces pallor, sweating, apprehension, weakness and even circumoral paraesthesiae. A blood glucose taken at the time of symptoms will confirm the diagnosis (< 2 mmol/l) and intravenous dextrose reverses the picture.

Ketotic diabetic coma usually has a slower onset and may be triggered by an intercurrent infection. Many patients appear ill, dehydrated with a dry skin, and often deep, rapid respirations—'air hunger'. The smell of acetone may be detected on their breath. Often there are complaints of abdominal pain, nausea and vomiting. Consciousness may be lost, usually without focal neurological signs, although tendon reflexes may be depressed. Another type of coma may be seen in diabetics, hyperosmolar non-ketotic: here there is severe dehydration, viscous blood, hypernatraemia but no ketosis. There is often severe potassium depletion.

Thiamine deficiency (page 122) may cause mental changes followed by a deteriorating conscious level. It is more common in chronic alcoholics. *Anoxia* may cause a depressed conscious level. This may arise after a cardiac arrest, follow cardiac surgery, or any situation decreasing cerebral perfusion.

In coma caused by poisoning, anoxia or of metabolic origin there is commonly a preceding deteriorating conscious level. Pupillary reactions, conjugate eye movements and brain stem functions are preserved at this stage. As deterioration occurs these may be lost. There may also be respiratory depression, Cheyne-Stokes breathing or altered respiratory patterns, particularly if acidosis has occurred. Motor disturbances include tremors (e.g. liver flap) and involuntary movements (e.g. anoxic myoclonus): motor signs in the limbs may be widespread or even focal (e.g. a hemiparesis). Most commonly the limbs withdraw symmetrically from painful stimuli, tone is reduced and the reflexes depressed, the plantar responses being extensor. Decerebrate posturing is a late feature.

In the neurological unit, the causes of coma are usually structurally determined (Table IV). In the elderly, strokes are very common but a fluctuating picture raises the possibility of a subdural haematoma. A progressive picture suggests an expanding mass from a tumour or even an abscess. Epileptic fits may cause loss of consciousness which may be prolonged if serial fits or status epilepticus has occurred. In the neurosurgical unit, patients with head injuries are common. Toxic ill patients may have a depressed conscious level from meningitis or encephalitis: this may not always be accompanied by fever.

Investigations: Preserve any containers brought by relatives or attendants in patients suspected of self-poisoning. A blood sample should be taken for an FBC, ESR, glucose, urea and electrolytes. A sample may also be necessary for liver function tests and an estimation of drug or alcohol levels. Under selected conditions certain other tests may be indicated — endocrine functions, blood pH, blood and urine osmolalities (where inappropriate secretion of antidiuretic hormone (ADH) is suspected). If an infective process is suspected, blood cultures should be made. A urine sample may be helpful for routine analysis, drug levels, osmolality and even porphyrins.

An EEG is a useful test when the conscious level is depressed. Often there is a widespread slow wave disturbance which is non-specific. However a focal disturbance may indicate a local structural lesion as an abscess or tumour. Certain rare encephalitic processes may show periodic widespread discharges which may be diagnostic e.g. herpes simplex encephalitis. Diffuse fast activity may suggest drug intoxication.

Plain X-rays of the skull and chest should be taken: the former may show features of raised ICP or trauma. A *CT brain scan* is the most useful test. In a truly comatose patient there is little problem with the procedure but the restless, confused, unco-operative patient may require a general anaesthetic (GA) to produce adequate quality pictures. When such procedures are not available carotid angiography may prove useful. This can show the presence of a supratentorial mass or hydrocephalus, the last suggesting a posterior fossa mass.

In patients where a mass lesion has been excluded or where intracranial infection or an SAH is suspected (particularly if there is meningism), the CSF should be examined. The pressure should be measured and samples taken for cytology, staining, culture and for chemical estimations. In patients where a mass is suspected it is better to defer the lumbar puncture until after the CT scan; this avoids risks of coning. In patients suspected of having an intracranial mass, particularly in the posterior fossa, and where the conscious level is depressed, it is wise to liaise at an early stage of the investigations with the neurosurgical team.

Treatment: this depends on the cause. During the investigations it is important that patients' signs are regularly monitored and charted so that changes can be followed. Such changes may necessitate specific therapy. If a mass is found then urgent neurosurgical advice should be sought. If no mass is demonstrated, appropriate support and management should be continued while a diagnosis is being made. Patients will require the maintenance of a clear airway, and regular turning and positioning. Fluid and caloric supplements should be given with added vitamins. These may need to be given initially by intravenous infusion or through a nasogastric tube. Catheterisation may be necessary and fluid balance charts should be kept.

6. THE RESPIRATORY UNIT OR INTENSIVE CARE UNIT (ICU)

Respiratory Failure

This indicates a defect preventing adequate oxygenation of the blood and elimination of carbon dioxide. Failure occurs when the arterial oxygen tension is less than 8.0 kPa (60 mm Hg) or if the carbon dioxide tension is above 6.6 kPa (50 mm Hg). The defect may arise in many ways:

1. Mechanical obstruction of the airway. This may be simple, e.g. mucus or vomit, or more severe from laryngeal oedema or spasm. Comatose patients may show signs of airway obstruction.

2. Upset of the 'bellows' may arise from weakness in the muscles of the diaphragm and rib cage, or from damage to the nerves that 'drive' these muscles. Acute neurogenic causes include polyneuritis, poliomyelitis and myasthenia gravis. Intense muscle spasm may interfere with respiration: this can occur in tetanus or with prolonged or serial epileptic fits. Rarely polymyositis and some myopathies may cause respiratory failure. Trauma with crush injuries to the chest may also be responsible.

More common causes of cardio-respiratory failure from lung and heart disease will not be discussed here.

Bulbar paralysis causes failure of the automatic reflexes protecting the airway from spill-over of food and oral secretions. Such patients aspirate these secretions leading acutely to tracheal or bronchial obstruction, or more slowly to the development of bronchopneumonia. In many instances, this is accompanied by depression or absence of the protective cough reflex. Damage within the lower brain stem cranial nerves (9, 10 and 12) produces a bulbar paralysis, e.g. polio, Coxsackie infections, polyneuritis, brain stem infarcts or demyelination, tumours and myasthenia gravis.

Many of the neural causes of respiratory disturbance also upset bulbar function.

Symptoms and signs: Conscious patients may complain of breathlessness or difficulty swallowing. With bulbar weakness, aspiration may occur when swallowing is attempted and this may provoke choking and coughing. Many such patients avoid drinking and may spit out saliva. Coughing may be weak and non-productive. Nasal regurgitation of fluids during drinking suggests paralysis of the soft palate. The voice may also be affected. Patients with impending respiratory failure may be anxious and restless; this is more likely to occur by the evening when they are tired. It is dangerous to sedate such patients.

Some patients appear cyanotic with rapid shallow respiration. Although various tests, as counting aloud in a single deep breath or blowing out a match, give a rough assessment of respiratory function, it is better to measure the vital capacity (VC) using one of the small portable spirometers. VC is the volume produced by a maximal inspiration followed by a maximal expiration. Normal values vary with age and sex but in adults when the VC falls to 1.0 l or less, a potentially dangerous situation has been reached. In severe neurogenic respiratory failure the VC may reach levels near that of the tidal volume. In making VC measurements it is important to prevent air leakage through the nose or an ill-fitting mask or mouth piece. This is common if patients have weak facial muscles.

Blood gas measurements (pH, Pco_2, and Po_2) are most useful. These together with a minute volume may be all the information available in unconscious patients.

In conscious patients, swallowing difficulties can be assessed by a test sip of water. In unconscious patients the presence of a 'gag' reflex indicates some airway protection but often secretions need regular suction. In deep coma the 'gag' is lost. Laryngoscopic examination of the upper airway may be possible and the mobility of the vocal cords assessed.

Treatment: With severe respiratory failure from neuromuscular causes it is necessary to overcome any bulbar weakness and provide effective artificial ventilation. With pure bulbar weakness a head down tilt of 15° allows secretions to run out of the mouth, aided by gravity. Adults and some children will not tolerate this position so it is necessary to protect the airway with a cuffed endotracheal tube. This may be inserted through the mouth, or if it has to remain in place for any time, through the nose which is more comfortable. Modern plastic tubes may be left in place for several days but if patients have longer lasting problems, a tracheostomy should be performed and the tube inserted through the stoma. Ideally this should be done as a definitive surgical procedure under GA based on appropriate assessment, not as an emergency in critically ill patients with obstructed airways.

Artificial ventilation is now provided by ventilators which deliver intermittent positive pressure through the tracheal tube. Conscious patients with intact neuromuscular respiratory mechanisms will often 'fight' the action of the ventilator but in most neurological patients with respiratory weakness, or in those treated with curare, this does not happen. If it does to a significant degree, muscle relaxants may be necessary.

In a few patients with more chronic neuromuscular diseases a cuirass or tank ventilator ('iron lung') may still be used. These are absolutely contraindicated in patients with bulbar disturbance as they will suck in any oral secretions to the lungs in the inspiratory phase.

Patients with a tracheostomy and artificial ventilation need special nursing and physiotherapy. Posturing of the chest, tappotage and regular suction of the airways are necessary. Most soft suction catheters passed through a tracheostomy tube enter the right main bronchus. An angled catheter may be necessary to suck out the left bronchus. Humidification of the inspired air in tracheostomised patients is beneficial.

The mortality of patients with bulbar and respiratory weakness occurs largely from (i) respiratory failure, (ii) secondary bronchopneumonia, and (iii) pulmonary embolism. Tracheostomy and artificial ventilation avoids the first, good physiotherapy much of the second, and the use of heparin (often subcutaneous) the third.

Acute Polyneuritis (Landry-Guillain-Barré)

Patients may develop an acute polyneuritis with progressive paralysis and sensory loss commonly starting in the feet and ascending proximally. The arms are usually affected and the cranial nerves may be involved. In about 50% there may be bilateral facial weakness, in c. 30% bulbar weakness and in c. 25% respiratory weakness. The autonomic nerves may be affected with sphincter upset and disorders of heart rate, blood pressure and sweating.

In most patients the disease reaches its peak within three weeks of onset so that if patients can be supported through the acute phase of the illness, most will make a good recovery. Early symptoms include distal sensory tingling and numbness accompanied by weakness. Rarely the weakness is more marked proximally. Headache, malaise and acute back pain may be early features. Less commonly confusion and meningism may be present. About two thirds of patients give a history of a preceding infective illness, often a viral upper respiratory tract upset.

The signs are those of weakness and sensory loss in the territories of the affected peripheral and cranial nerves. In virtually all patients the reflexes are depressed or absent (the ankle jerks are always absent). Very rarely the plantar responses may be extensor. If there are symptoms and signs of significant bulbar and respiratory involvement it is wise to perform an elective tracheostomy.

Investigations: in 90% the CSF protein is elevated (> 0.5 g/l), sometimes very high. Occasionally the protein rise occurs later in the illness. The CSF gamma globulin fraction is commonly raised. Early reports suggested there was no CSF pleocytosis (2% had a lymphocytosis $> 15/mm^3$); however higher values have been found in serial CSF studies.

Nerve conduction studies commonly show marked slowing suggestive of demyelination in peripheral nerve fibres. Rarely there may be conduction block and in some patients, after two to three weeks, some fibrillation may be found. Changes may not appear in the first few days; commonly the clinical findings antedate the electrophysiological results and this lag is also seen during the recovery phase.

Paired sera for viral studies, a Paul Bunnell test and urine sample for porphyrins should be sent.

Treatment: involves appropriate nursing care and physiotherapy through the acute paralytic phase with artificial ventilation and a tracheostomy when there is significant bulbar and respiratory involvement. The autonomic upset may necessitate catheterisation, treatment for constipation, and special care if a labile blood pressure or arrhythmias appear. Many patients have been treated with high dose steroids but a recent controlled trial (Hughes *et al.*, 1978) showed no significant benefit in the treated group.

Tetanus

Tetanus is caused by the release of toxin from the anaerobe *Clostridium tetani*. By appropriate immunisation the disease can largely be prevented for an infected wound is the commonest source. In patients with a short incubation period, < 10 days, or a short duration from the first symptom to spasm, < 3 days, a severe form of the disease may appear.

The toxin causes paroxysmal muscle spasms triggered by any afferent stimulus so that bulbar disturbance (dysphagia) and respiratory spasm with prolonged apnoea appear.

Presenting symptoms include malaise, fever, headache, irritability and sweating. Stiffness of the jaw muscles (trismus) and the inability to open the mouth wide produces the risus sardonicus. Dysphagia and complaints of sore throat are common: patients dislike swallowing as this may provoke spasms which in turn cause choking and coughing. More severe spasms arch the body into opisthotonus with respiratory arrest and cyanosis. On relaxation of such a spasm there may be inhalation of pooled pharyngeal secretions which may trigger a further spasm. The muscles are stiff; the abdomen may even show board-like rigidity.

The sympathetic nervous system may be involved causing a labile blood pressure, the development of arrhythmias, severe sweating and even hyperpyrexia. Rarely patients may present with cephalic tetanus with cranial nerve palsies.

The diagnosis is *clinical*.

Treatment: in severe tetanus a tracheostomy is necessary so that patients can be paralysed with curare and artificially ventilated until the spasms wear off, often within two to three weeks. Tubocurarine (15 mg) or pancuronium (0.03–0.06 mg/kg) are relaxants commonly used. These are injected intramuscularly (IM) and staff are taught to give the next injection when the effect of the last has started to wear off (this may be every two hours in severely ill patients). In addition patients are commonly given intravenous diazepam by slow infusion (3–20 mg/kg/day) which helps to reduce the spasms and rigidity.

It is dangerous to attempt to pass a nasogastric tube in untreated patients with severe tetanus as this may provoke spasms. Any such tube should be passed after they have been intubated and 'curarised'.

In most patients, to avoid the complications of sympathetic involvement, alpha and beta blockers are given e.g. phenoxybenzamine and propranolol. Subcutaneous heparin (5000 units b.d) may be given to prevent pulmonary emboli.

Moderately ill patients, with dysphagia, trismus and moderate spasms, may be managed by tracheostomy and similar large doses of intravenous diazepam alone may be sufficient.

Any potentially infected wounds should be widely excised and a course of penicillin given for seven days. Anti-tetanus serum (ATS) has largely been replaced by human anti-tetanus immunoglobulin (Humotet); if available 1000–4000 units IM should be given. Patients who have already been immunised should receive a booster dose of toxoid.

Poliomyelitis

The polio virus is usually ingested and in unimmunised patients may produce a subclinical upset or prodromal illness. In the latter fever, malaise, sore throat or gastro-intestinal upset lasting one to two days are the most common. A proportion of such patients may then develop a meningitic or 'pre-paralytic' illness with intense headache, fever, vomiting and neck stiffness. Pains may also appear in the back and limbs.

In a small number of patients the paralytic phase develops with increasing muscle pain and paralysis. The paralysis is of lower motor neurone type with flaccid muscles, absent reflexes and there is no sensory loss. Paralysis is usually apparent within 2–5 days of the onset of the meningeal symptoms. It is often asymmetrical and may involve bulbar and respiratory muscles. Exercise in the early part of the illness should be avoided as it may cause the paralysis to extend.

Investigation: the CSF shows a pleocytosis in the meningitic phase, initially polymorphs and lymphocytes, later lymphocytes. The protein is elevated and the glucose normal. Viral CSF cultures are often sterile. The virus may be isolated from throat swabs or stool cultures. Paired sera (14–21 days apart) may show a rise in antibody titre.

Treatment: this is an infective illness so patients should be barrier nursed or isolated for three weeks. Bulbar and respiratory paralysis may require tracheostomy and artificial ventilation. In a proportion of affected patients, paralysed and weakened muscles may slowly recover and the number of patients left dependent on a permanent ventilator is small. Physiotherapy and rehabilitation play a major role in recovery.

Myasthenia Gravis (see page 119)

A few patients with generalised myasthenia have such severe weakness that bulbar and respiratory functions are dangerously compromised. Most of these patients have prominent proximal limb muscle weakness with involvement of ocular, facial and neck muscles. In known myasthenic patients sudden deterioration, a myasthenic crisis, may be due to a number of causes—infections (commonly respiratory), underdosage with anticholinesterases, or the use of certain drugs (e.g. curare, streptomycin, gentamicin). Occasionally undiagnosed myasthenic patients may present with respiratory failure, often with co-existent infection.

In a few patients with myasthenia receiving treatment with anti-cholinesterases (pyridostigmine, neostigmine) overdosage may occur, a cholinergic crisis. Here further treatment with these drugs will cause increased weakness.

To differentiate between a myasthenic and cholinergic crisis an *edrophonium (Tensilon)* test is necessary. Edrophonium is a short acting cholinesterase inhibitor which, when given IV, will cause an increase in strength in a myasthenic crisis, but a decrease in a cholinergic crisis. A test dose of 2 mg is usually given and after a pause to observe its effect, the remaining 8 mg are given. It is important to have an objective sign to follow e.g. ptosis, restricted eye movement, measured limb strength or swallowing ability. Most patients in a cholinergic crisis will also have constricted pupils unless atropine has been given.

Patients with severe bulbar or respiratory muscle weakness should be intubated and if necessary, artificially ventilated. In many patients if the deterioration is only of a few days duration, management may be possible with an endotracheal tube.

In patients with a myasthenic crisis an increased dose of anticholinesterase will be necessary. If patients cannot swallow, neostigmine can be given by IM injection (15 mg orally is equivalent to 1 mg IM). Most patients receiving a high dose of anticholinesterase will also need atropine (0.6 mg 8 hourly) to prevent diarrhoea, and decrease bronchial secretions and salivation. Other forms of treatment may need consideration, e.g. steroids. Some myasthenic patients who are being ventilated show a better response to their anticholinesterases if these are transiently stopped and then restarted.

In a cholinergic crisis very weak patients may need intubation, ventilation and atropine until the excess anticholinesterases have worn off.

Status Epilepticus

This is an emergency with a significant mortality and morbidity so it is essential to control the fits as soon as possible. If patients develop serial major fits, one attack following the last without recovery of consciousness, or they have a prolonged clonic phase, lasting more than 30 minutes, they are in danger.

In most patients convulsing can be temporarily stopped by the slow IV injection of diazepam (10 mg) or clonazepam (1 mg). Clonazepam is about ten times stronger than diazepam and more effective. However in many patients, the fits may recur so that it is wise to set up an IV infusion, preferably choosing a site where further fits will not dislodge the needle. Patients' airways should also be protected. Patients then may be transferred to an ICU where facilities for monitoring their progress and for intubation and ventilation, if necessary, are available.

Many different regimes are used to control fits. In all the airway should be secured. It should also be noted that many patients may already have received a number of anticonvulsants which may have caused respiratory or cardiovascular depression, so that further anticonvulsant treatment may prove cumulative. To control the fits IV infusions include:

1. Clonazepam, 3 mg in 250 ml of normal saline (usually 1–3 mg in 6 hours is effective),
2. Diazepam, 50–100 mg in 500 ml of normal saline,
3. Chlormethiazole in a 0.8% solution infused at rates of 0.5–0.7 g/hour,
4. Thiopentone sodium, 1.0 g in 500 ml of Ringer lactate (usually c. 1.0 g in 12 hours),
5. Phenytoin sodium, 100–200 mg given slowly, which may need repetition.

These are all adult doses.

In all instances the infusion is started rapidly to stop the fits, and the rate then reduced to control the attacks. While being controlled, attention should be turned to the cause for the status, and to the establishment of an effective oral anticonvulsant regimen. A blood sample taken on admission to measure patients' anticonvulsant levels, may prove most useful in establishing underdosage or non-compliance as causes for the status.

Other neurological patients may be nursed in the ICU if critically ill with meningitis, encephalitis, head injury or SAH. Some post-operative patients and a few with other disorders may be included. In all patients the emphasis is on regular continued observation, specialised nursing care, and the availability of the rapid and effective means of treating acute respiratory or bulbar failure.

7. INFECTIONS

Meningitis

The commonest infection of the nervous system is meningitis where the leptomeninges may be invaded by bacteria, viruses or rarely fungi. Symptoms of *meningeal irritation, meningism,* include headache, nausea and vomiting, photophobia, irritability, drowsiness and confusion. Complaints may be made of pain in the neck and back, and of malaise. In more severely affected patients there may be a deteriorating conscious level and patients may present in coma, with a fit or with focal neurological disturbance.

The signs of *meningism* are neck stiffness and reduced straight leg raising (Kernig's sign). These are accompanied by fever. Often patients lie flexed in a 'ball', resentful of light or interference. Complications may arise: a thrombotic endarteritis may produce focal neurological signs and isolated cranial nerve palsies may appear. In infants with meningitis, the anterior fontanelle may be tense.

In the very young and sometimes the very old, meningism may be absent or minimal. Patients with poor defences e.g. with leukaemia, or on treatment with steroids or immunosuppressive drugs, may develop meningitis with fever and only minimal signs.

Many patients have raised intracranial pressure and some papilloedema. However a stiff neck and papilloedema may also be produced by a pressure cone from a mass, particularly in the posterior fossa: here a lumbar puncture may prove dangerous. Papilloedema with meningism may also occur with intracranial infections—cerebral abscess, subdural empyema, cortical thrombophlebitis or major venous sinus thrombosis. In all such instances an *urgent CT scan* should be performed to exclude a mass before patients have a lumbar puncture.

Diagnosis of meningitis is made from the CSF. This should be examined microscopically and cultures set up. It is important to alert the laboratory staff if a tuberculous (TB) or fungal infection is suspected. A CSF sample in a fluoride bottle for glucose estimation should always be sent, and a blood glucose sample taken at the same time. Blood cultures should be taken; these may prove positive when CSF cultures are sterile. An FBC, ESR, urea and electrolytes, and X-rays of the skull and chest should be included. If viral infections are suspected, cultures should be made from throat swabs and stools. Paired sera may be sent to test for any rise in antibody levels. Unfortunately many patients may have received an antibiotic before admission which may render CSF cultures sterile.

Bacterial Meningitis

Bacterial infections are much more dangerous with an appreciable mortality and morbidity. These increase the longer treatment is delayed. Common causes are from the meningococcus, pneumococcus and *Haemophilus influenzae*. The last is more common in children under six. In neonates a number of other organisms may be responsible—the staphylococcus, streptococcus or *Escherichia coli*.

Patients with meningococcal and pneumococcal infections may be critically ill. With meningococcal infections there may be a widespread petechial rash (c. 30%), a purpuric rash or even septicaemic shock. The Waterhouse-Friderichsen syndrome describes patients with meningococcal septicaemia in acute shock who have bilateral suprarenal haemorrhages usually as part of a widespread haemorrhagic tendency. Other complications include the development of cranial nerve palsies (3, 6, 7 & 8), fits, subdural effusions, hydrocephalus and disseminated intravascular coagulopathy (DIC). Herpetic lesions on the lips are common. Epidemics may occur.

The CSF appears turbid (purulent) and is often under pressure. There is a polymorph leucocytosis, $500–3000 + /mm^3$, an elevated protein, 1.0–3.0 g/l, and a very low glucose. The CSF lactate is usually > 3.3 mmol/l. Stains may show intra- and extracellular Gram-negative diplococci. Recent studies on the CSF with countercurrent immunoelectrophoresis enables detection of meningococcal antigen. Positive blood cultures are common.

Treatment: large doses of intravenous benzyl penicillin best given as bolus doses four hourly into a running drip. In adults 2–3 mega-units (1.2–1.8 g) given four hourly; in children the dose is 250 000 units (0.15 g)/kg/day. This can be combined with a sulphonamide, e.g. sulphadiazine 100 mg/kg/day given in divided doses six hourly. About 10% of meningococci are sulphonamide resistant. Chloramphenicol, 2–4 g/day in adults, given in divided doses is another useful drug with good entry into the CSF and which can be used in patients with a history of penicillin-allergy.

As recovery occurs, the blood-brain barrier becomes more impermeable to drugs so that at a time when patients are improving a lower dose may be reaching the CSF. Thus it is important not to reduce the dose too soon. The duration of treatment is usually 7–10 days but is determined by patients' progress.

Pneumococcal meningitis often occurs in older patients with spread of infection from the lungs, middle ear or sinuses. In the elderly there is a high mortality (25%). The CSF shows similar findings to a meningococcal infection but stains may show Gram positive diplococci. Pneumococcal antigen can also be identified by CSF immuno-electrophoresis. Positive blood cultures are common. Treatment is with high doses of IV penicillin as for meningococcal infections, continued for at least 10 days. Chloramphenicol is also effective.

Haemophilus meningitis is commonest in children and often secondary to a respiratory infection. The onset may be more insidious with children that are fretful and drowsy. The CSF findings are similar to other bacterial infections but stains show Gram negative bacilli. Treatment is with chloramphenicol, 4 g/day in adults, and 50–100 mg/kg/day in children, in divided doses for 10 days. High dose ampicillin, 300–400 mg/kg/day, given in divided bolus doses IV, is also effective but some resistant organisms have been reported and ampicillin may produce a sensitivity rash.

Tuberculous Meningitis

Tuberculous meningitis (TBM) is now rare. It is more common in immigrants. Again delay in diagnosis and treatment increases the mortality and morbidity. Often the early symptoms are rather non-specific—malaise, apathy, anorexia and a low grade fever. Many patients but not all have headache and vomiting although these may appear later. Patients diagnosed later are often drowsy, may have fits, neurological signs, cranial nerve palsies and even papilloedema. The build up of the illness may have taken a few weeks rather than days.

The CSF findings may be variable. Commonly there is an elevated lymphocyte count, up to $400/mm^3$, a high protein, 1.0–6.0 g/l, and a low glucose < 2.2 mmol/l. The lactate is usually > 3.3 mmol/l. Finding tubercle bacilli in the CSF confirms the diagnosis but cultures or animal inoculation may take three or more weeks to become positive. Repeated CSF examinations may give an answer but occasional patients are reported with normal CSF findings. A bromide partition test (page 23) may show the ratio of bromide in the blood : CSF to be less than 1.6. Other helpful tests include; chest X-ray (positive in c. 70%), and tuberculin test (Mantoux 1 : 100 positive in c. 78%). Skull X-rays and CT scans may show intracranial calcification, tuberculomas or even hydrocephalus.

Treatment schedules vary. Most patients receive three or four drugs initially. When the results of cultures and sensitivities are available then the drugs may be modified. Treatment should include; (i) isoniazid (INAH)—10–15 mg/kg/day. This enters the CSF well. Occasionally it produces a polyneuritis and to prevent this pyridoxine, 10-40 mg/day, should be added. (ii) rifampicin—10 mg/kg/day or 600 mg/day, given in a single oral dose is another effective drug although it does not enter the CSF well. It may cause abnormal liver function tests. To these may be added (iii) pyrazinamide—20-40 mg/kg/day to a total of 3 g/day, given orally in three divided doses. This has good CSF penetration but may cause liver damage or precipitate gout. Alternatively for (iii) streptomycin—1.0 g/day IM may be used. In the elderly and those with renal damage the dose should be lowered. It does not enter the CSF well and may be given intrathecally, 50 mg/day for one week and then on alternate days for two weeks. The chief toxic effect is on the eighth cranial nerve. This can be combined with ethambutol—25–35 mg/kg/day, given as a single oral dose. It enters the CSF less well and with prolonged use may produce a toxic optic neuritis. Usually streptomycin and ethambutol are used for only three months, but INAH, and rifampicin for at least twelve months. Pyrazinamide may be continued for twelve months too.

There is debate about the use of steroids. They may be helpful in preventing the development of a spinal block. Evidence that their use reduces mortality and morbidity is conflicting.

Non-bacterial Meningitis

In some patients the *CSF may show a pleocytosis*, often *lymphocytic*, a mildly elevated protein and a normal or slightly depressed glucose. Stains including those for acid-fast bacilli, show no bacteria, cultures are sterile and the patient appears ill. The differential diagnosis includes:

1. Viral meningitis
2. TBM
3. Leptospiral meningitis
4. Fungal meningitis
5. Syphilis
6. Sarcoidosis
7. Thrombophlebitis, or venous sinus thrombosis
8. Subdural empyema
9. Cerebral abscess
10. Partially treated pyogenic meningitis.

Viral infections are common (Table V), often mumps, Coxsackie or Echo

Table V
Neurological Infections

Meningitis (common forms)		
Bacterial	Meningococcus	
	Pneumococcus	
	Haemophilus influenzae	
	Escherichia coli }	
	Streptococcus }	Neonates
	Staphylococcus }	
Viral	Mumps }	
	Coxsackie }	may be a meningo-encephalitis
	Echovirus }	
Fungal	*Cryptococcus neoformans*	(rare)
Neoplastic		
Encephalitis		
Enteroviruses	Coxsackie }	
	Echo }	(rare)
	Polio }	
Arthropod-borne	Equine }	(very rare in GB)
	Japanese B }	
Sporadic	Herpes simplex	
	Mumps	
	Herpes zoster	
	Rabies	
Post-infective	Post-vaccination	
	Measles, Rubella, Varicella, Glandular Fever, 'Flu	
Subacute Sclerosing Pan-encephalitis (SSPE)		

virus. Patients are usually not severely ill. The CSF shows a raised white cell count, 50–500/mm³, predominantly lymphocytes. The protein is often elevated, 0.5–1.0 g/l, and the glucose usually normal. Rarely the glucose is low. The CSF lactate is usually < 2.8 mmol/l. Some other conditions may produce similar CSF changes (page 47). Viral infections commonly have a good prognosis and only require supportive treatment.

Leptospiral meningitis is a rare infection. Most patients have associated liver and renal upset. A polymorph leucocytosis in the blood and albuminuria are usual. There is a raised agglutination titre in the serum and the organism may be identified in the blood and urine. Treatment is with penicillin.

Fungal meningitis is also rare. The most common organism is the cryptococcus and it occurs more frequently in patients with damaged defences. Special CSF stains and cultures may give the diagnosis. A cryptococcal antigen may be detected in the blood and CSF. The organism is often hard to eliminate but IV amphotericin B (20 mg/day) and oral flucytosine (150 mg/kg/day), given together in a six week course, are often successful.

Partially treated meningitis: if this is suspected, counter-current immuno-electrophoresis of the CSF may help identify some of the pyogenic causes. Where the cause is uncertain and probably bacterial, chloramphenicol is a most useful antibiotic.

Intracranial thrombophlebitis and *venous sinus thrombosis* may follow meningitis and local infections. Head injuries, severe anaemia, dehydration, or changes in blood coagulability—the last being common post-partum, may be causes. Usually there are symptoms and signs of raised ICP, focal signs (depending on the site) and fits. CT scanning and/or angiography may establish the diagnosis. Treatment depends on the cause but includes antibiotics if infective. Steroids may be used to reduce cerebral oedema and anticonvulsants to control fits. Anticoagulants are contra-indicated.

Subdural Empyema

This may result from the spread of infection from the frontal sinuses or mastoids. It may occur in children with meningitis. Pus collects and spreads over the surface of one hemisphere which may be irritated and compressed: this may cause fits or focal signs (e.g. contralateral hemiparesis), and elevated ICP. Plain skull X-rays may show the source of infection, and a CT scan the empyema, although sometimes these may appear isodense. Treatment is by surgical drainage and antibiotics. If there is a high clinical suspicion of a collection then a burr-hole should be made. Some subdural empyemas lead to a secondary venous thrombosis.

Cerebral Abscess

This is a life-threatening condition with an appreciable mortality despite treatment. Infection commonly spreads from local structures as the middle ear, sinuses, from penetrating scalp wounds, dental sepsis or may be blood-borne. In the last group the site may arise from bacterial endocarditis, intrathoracic sepsis or cyanotic congenital heart disease. General symptoms of infection may be minimal, depending on the origin of the sepsis. Usually there are features of raised ICP accompanied by fever and focal signs. Fits may be the presenting symptom. The signs depend on the abscess site. Middle ear and mastoid sepsis tend to produce temporal lobe or cerebellar abscesses, paranasal sinus sepsis spreads to the frontal lobes. Haematogenous spread may produce multiple abscesses at different sites, usually supratentorial.

Investigations: FBC, ESR and blood cultures may be helpful. Skull and chest X-rays, and EEG and CT scan with enhancement (Plates 7, 8) should be done. The last gives a definitive answer. Isotope scans and angiography may show an abscess. Lumbar puncture is contra-indicated as it may produce a pressure cone.

Treatment: by surgical evacuation together with large doses of systemic antibiotics. Surgeons may use a burr-hole and aspiration or total excision. Antibiotics may be instilled into the abscess cavity and sometimes radio-opaque contrast to follow progress. Many abscesses contain unusual organisms; *Strep. milleri, Bacteroides fragilis* and *Staph. aureus* are the most common. In otogenic cerebral abscesses Proteus and Bacteroides are common—the last is an anaerobe. Antibiotics should include (i) ampicillin and flucloxacillin (4 g/day of each), (ii) gentamicin (80 mg 8 hourly) and (iii) metronidazole (400–600 mg 8 hourly). The last destroys anaerobes. This combination may be used to start treatment until the results of cultures and sensitivities are available. The source of infection may also need treatment. Steroids may be used to reduce surrounding oedema. There is a high incidence of epilepsy following an abscess so anticonvulsants should be started.

Encephalitis

This is rare. The most usual form is viral meningo-encephalitis and in Britain herpes simplex is the commonest cause of encephalitis.

The onset is often acute with headache, prostration, fever and sometimes meningism—the last depending on the degree of meningeal involvement. This may be negligible. As the brain becomes progressively involved and swells there is a deteriorating conscious level which may proceed to coma. Fits are very common. Focal signs or those of diffuse neurological disturbance appear. Certain infections show a predilection for one site e.g. the temporal lobes in herpes simplex. Occasionally the presenting symptoms may be largely psychiatric.

Investigations: CSF may show a lymphocytic pleocytosis, a mild protein rise and normal glucose. Red cells may be present in herpes simplex infections. The CSF may be normal. The EEG is usually diffusely abnormal and may prove diagnostic. Repetitive periodic discharges are often seen in herpes simplex. A CT scan may be unremarkable or show patchy areas of low density—areas of necrosis. Areas of haemorrhage may appear as high density lesions and are often seen in herpes simplex. Viruses may be isolated from stools or throat swabs, and paired sera may show a rise in antibody titre. The place for brain biopsy is debated: this may afford a diagnosis particularly if electron microscopy is also undertaken, but as at present there is no known effective anti-viral chemotherapy, this invasive procedure needs justification.

Treatment: largely symptomatic and supportive. Steroids (dexamethasone 5 mg IM every six hours) initially in high dose, and then tapering off, may be used to reduce cerebral oedema. Trials using idoxyuridine and cytosine arabinoside have not shown consistent proven benefit. Acycloguanosine is under trial. Recovery may follow but in severely affected patients there is an appreciable mortality and morbidity.

Herpes Zoster (Shingles)

This is an acute viral infection of the first sensory neurone of spinal roots or cranial nerves. The virus is similar to varicella. Rarely the infection is symptomatic—secondary to a carcinoma or tumour at the affected level of the spinal root, or may follow trauma or even systemic infection. The incubation is 7–24 days, usually about 14 days.

Pain accompanied by malaise and fever is the presentation. The pain is in the distribution of the dermatomes of the affected roots and usually occurs three to four days before the appearance of the classical eruption, which confirms the diagnosis. The CSF commonly shows a mild lymphocytic pleocytosis, mild protein rise and normal glucose. The main complications are:

1. Post-herpetic neuralgia—occurs in c. 15%, particularly solitary, elderly patients. It produces persistent pain and discomfort notoriously difficult to treat. Analgesics, antidepressants, topical preparations and electrical stimulation in affected areas are used to try and alleviate the discomfort.

2. Ophthalmic zoster—trigeminal ganglion involvement with eruption over the forehead and inflammation of the eye. The cornea may be scarred, the lids and conjunctiva severely swollen, and less commonly actual oculomotor pareses and optic nerve involvement may occur. Needs urgent treatment to the eye—ophthalmic referral, the use of local steroids, antibiotics and acetazolamide to reduce intra-ocular pressure.

3. Geniculate zoster (Ramsay Hunt syndrome)—geniculate ganglion involved. Vesicles may be seen in the external ear with the development of a severe LMN facial palsy with loss of taste in the anterior two thirds of the tongue on the same side. The eighth nerve may be involved with acute vertigo and deafness.

4. Muscle wasting and weakness may be seen in a segmental distribution in affected areas—very rare.
5. Sphincter upset—sacral nerves may be involved with sphincter disturbance e.g. retention. Vesicles may be seen in the bladder at cystoscopy.
6. Meningo-encephalitis and myelitis—very rare.

Syphilis

Spirochaetal infection of the central nervous system by *Treponema pallidum* is now rare. To exclude unusual presentations specific serological tests should be undertaken e.g. TPHA, FTA(Abs).

Serological tests: non-specific or lipoidal tests include the Wassermann (WR), the Venereal Disease Research Laboratory (VDRL), Rapid Plasma Reagin (RPR) and Automated Reagin (ART). The drawbacks to these are that a small number of patients with neurosyphilis may have a negative test and occasionally false positives may occur e.g. after acute infection or in connective tissue disorders.

Specific tests include Reiter Protein Complement Fixation (RPCFT), Fluorescent Treponemal Antibody (absorbed)—FTA(Abs), Treponemal Haemagglutination (TPHA) and Treponemal Immobilisation (TPI). These use treponemal antigen and are more reliable. They are positive if infection has occurred: they seldom change with treatment. High levels of anti-treponemal antibody, IgM, in the CSF usually indicates active neurosyphilis.

In *secondary syphilis* about 2% of patients show acute meningism. Such patients may be unwell, febrile, have muscle pains, a maculo-papular skin rash, enlarged lymph nodes and often ulcers on mucosal surfaces. Microscopic examination of sera from these ulcers may show spirochaetes. In the CSF there is commonly a lymphocytic pleocytosis, mild protein rise and normal glucose. Serological blood tests are usually positive.

Treatment: in all forms of syphilis this is with penicillin—600 000 units of procaine penicillin injected daily IM for 21 days. Erythromycin or tetracycline (2 g/day) for 21 days may be used in patients with penicillin-allergy.

Late syphilis

This occurs often 5–10 years after infection.

1. Meningovascular or Cerebrospinal Syphilis

a. Cerebral involvement   (i) leptomeningeal—usually present with headache, memory impairment, anxiety, fits. Abnormal pupillary reactions and cranial nerve palsies are common.

(ii) thrombotic endarteritis—usually present with an 'acute stroke' e.g. a hemiplegia.

(iii) gumma—very rare; presents as a mass.

b. Spinal involvement

(i) pachymeningitis—myelopathy (Erb's spastic paraplegia) affecting the cervical cord. Pain with wasting and weakness in hand and arm muscles, accompanied by a spastic paraplegia and sphincter upset.

(ii) thrombotic endarteritis of spinal cord vessels—acute myelopathy.

CSF usually abnormal with increased lymphocytes and protein. Serology in blood and CSF usually positive with specific tests; non-specific blood tests are positive in c. 70%.

2. Parenchymal Involvement—usually 8–10 years after injection.

Tabes dorsalis (Locomotor ataxia); here there is a loss of the dorsal columns. Presents with lightning pains and paraesthesiae, commonly in the legs accompanied by unsteadiness. Patients show marked sensory ataxia with loss of posterior column and deep pain sensation. The last may lead to neuropathic ulcers, often perforating, on the soles, and neuropathic joints (Charcot's)—painless, disorganised weight-bearing joints. Crises with acute pain may occur e.g. gastric, rectal. Reflexes are depressed or lost, 90% show Argyll Robertson pupils (light-near dissociation) and some optic atrophy and ptosis. Sphincter upsets are common with a large atonic bladder causing overflow incontinence; c. 20% have tabo-paresis where the plantar responses may be extensor.

General Paralysis of the Insane (GPI). These patients present with a progressive dementia; a few still show the florid delusions of grandeur. Behavioural changes are common. Later there is physical deterioration with fits (c. 50%), slurred speech, tremors of the face, lips and tongue, and of the hands. Incontinence, clumsiness and the appearance of cortico-spinal tract signs, usually bilateral appear later. Argyll Robertson pupils are common. CSF is abnormal, usually with a mild pleocytosis and elevated protein. The blood and CSF serological (specific) tests are usually positive.

Treatment: in all these forms, there may occasionally be a deterioration due to a Jarisch-Herxheimer reaction when penicillin treatment is started. If there is an associated syphilitic aortitis this may be potentially dangerous. For these reasons treatment with penicillin is often preceded by a short course of steroids—prednisolone 40 mg daily for two days and then 20 mg daily for three days, starting the penicillin injections on day two.

8. CEREBROVASCULAR DISEASE

An acute stroke describes an area of brain damage from circulatory disturbance. If this damage has left persisting signs, a completed stroke has occurred. The disturbance of circulation may arise from haemorrhage, most common in hypertensive patients, from embolism, usually from the heart or roughened extra-cranial arterial surfaces, or from thrombotic occlusion. The symptoms and signs produced, depend in part on the site and extent of damage.

A 'stroke in evolution' or 'continuing stroke' describes the slow development of clinical deficit often in a step-wise fashion over several hours. This progression may last as long as one to two days and when it has reached its peak a completed stroke has occurred. 'Continuing strokes' raise diagnostic difficulties: is the deterioration due to an expanding haematoma, abscess or tumour, or to an extending infarct or the development of cerebral oedema?

Transient ischaemic attacks (TIAs) are brief episodes of focal neurological disturbance with an abrupt onset. Usually there is full recovery within several minutes: most doctors accept a duration of up to 24 hours but if they last longer a stroke has occurred. TIAs may herald the onset of a devastating stroke.

Acute Strokes

These patients present with focal neurological deficits, commonly a hemiplegia. *Embolism* has the most rapid onset, often with preservation of consciousness. Confusion, fits and headache may occur and the deficit is often complete from the onset. Embolic infarction has a higher incidence than previously suspected. Emboli may arise from the heart—from diseased valves, mural thrombus over a myocardial infarct or thrombus in an atrial appendage. Other major embolic sources are atheromatous ulcers or stenotic areas in the extracranial feeding arteries.

Haemorrhagic infarction may have a rapid onset often with progressive deficit appearing over a few minutes. Exertion or emotion may precipitate a bleed. Many patients are hypertensive. Headache and vomiting are common and there may be a deteriorating conscious level leading to coma. If blood enters the CSF, meningism will be present.

Cerebral infarction from *thrombotic occlusion* of a vessel is common. The onset is usually more gradual sometimes starting with rather non-specific symptoms as dizziness or headache. Focal deficit appears early and may progress. Consciousness is commonly preserved at the onset but oedema may develop around an infarct causing deterioration. However such deterioration may be due to other causes e.g. bronchopneumonia.

The site and extent of the area of infarction will produce differing signs. More posteriorly placed hemisphere lesions may cause a contralateral hemisensory disturbance or hemianopia. More anteriorly placed lesions produce a hemiplegia. Dominant hemisphere involvement produces dysphasia. If the frontal eye field is damaged then there may be tonic deviation of the head and eyes towards the affected frontal lobe i.e. away from the side of the hemiplegic limbs. Infarcts within the brain stem arise from lesions in the vertebrobasilar (VB) arteries or their branches. More remote damage involves the occipital cortex with the appearance of field defects. Within the *brain stem* three main arterial branches can be involved producing clear cut signs although some overlap may occur. All cause ipsilateral cerebellar upset and a Horner's syndrome, often with vertigo and vomiting at the onset. The lowest branch, the *posterior inferior cerebellar artery*, also causes ipsilateral spinothalamic sensory upset in the face, dysphagia and dysphonia (CN 9 & 10). On the contralateral side there is spinothalamic sensory loss on the trunk and limbs and occasionally a hemiparesis. The highest branch, *the superior cerebellar artery,* may produce ipsilateral deafness and choreic involuntary movements in addition to the cerebellar upset. Spinothalamic sensory upset of the face, trunk and limbs is all contralateral. Between these there is an area supplied by the *anterior inferior cerebellar artery*, which causes ipsilateral spinothalamic facial upset, an ipsilateral LMN facial weakness, deafness (CN 7 & 8) and contralateral spinothalamic loss in the limbs and trunk. *High lesions* in the brain stem may produce a hemiplegia with impaired conjugate gaze and deviation of the eyes towards the hemiplegic limbs.

Management

In acute stroke:
1. Secure airway and place in appropriate nursing position.
2. Assessment—conscious level, neurological signs, pupillary reactions and eye movement.
3. Cardio-pulmonary function assessed.

These allow a baseline so progress can be monitored. Deterioration may indicate airway obstruction, development of bronchopneumonia or heart failure, increasing cerebral oedema, an expanding haematoma, or an alternative diagnosis e.g. infection or tumour.

Investigations: in only two thirds of stroke patients is the pathogenesis correct at the bedside. In many the anatomical diagnosis is wrong and about 5% of patients have tumours not strokes.

1. Blood sample—FBC, ESR, urea, electrolytes, glucose, lipids and WR.
2. Cardiac function—ECG. If paroxysmal changes are suspected then 24 hour monitoring with a portable ECG may be necessary. Some patients with acute strokes or SAHs show ECG changes—T wave flattening and inversion, a prolonged QT interval and ST depression.
3. X-rays of the chest and skull.
4. CT scan—not always necessary but allows accurate exclusion of other pathology. Blood shows clearly as a high density lesion (Plate 10) and areas of infarction as low density sites (Plate 9b). Appearances may alter in the first few days after an infarct and very small areas may be difficult to show.
5. Isotope scan—may show an infarct, particularly supratentorial. In the first seven days some scans may appear negative. In positive scans caused by an infarct, there is often resolution if the scan is repeated after six to eight weeks. Isotope scans are less accurate and do not differentiate haemorrhagic from thrombo-embolic infarction.
6. EEG—may show a localised slow wave abnormality at a site of infarction. Serial studies may show improvement.
7. Angiography—seldom indicated in an acute stroke. It may show an occluded vessel or 'mass' but in many patients appears 'normal'. Some patients may deteriorate after angiography and it seldom influences management except to exclude other pathology. In an acute stroke the demonstration of an occluded vessel or tight stenosis is not usually followed by urgent surgical treatment.
8. CSF examination—essential if meningitis or haemorrhage needs exclusion. In a bleed, the CSF will appear blood-stained and the supernatant xanthochromic. In about 15% of patients where a cerebral haemorrhage has occurred within the brain tissue, the CSF may be clear. After thrombo-embolic infarction the CSF may appear normal but in many instances there may be a mild protein rise and occasionally a pleocytosis, commonly lymphocytic. In many patients only some of these investigations are indicated (or are available).

Treatment: *Chest and airway*—a depressed conscious level or brain stem damage with bulbar paresis may cause airway obstruction. Here an airway, regular turning, positioning and suction with chest physiotherapy are necessary.

Blood pressure and circulation—some patients show an elevated BP. This may be reactive or sustained; with the latter there are usually retinal changes, an enlarged heart, ECG changes or even albuminuria. A persistent high BP in younger patients (> 110 mm Hg diastolic) after 24–48 hours needs lowering to a level of c. 90 mm Hg. In elderly patients only very high levels of pressure need a slow reduction by treatment. A persistently high diastolic pressure of > 130 mm Hg requires more urgent treatment.

Cerebral vasodilators have not proved beneficial in an acute stroke. Cerebral blood flow studies show a fall in areas of infarction. The autoregulation of flow to such areas is impaired or lost and even CO_2 inhalation, a most potent vasodilator, appears ineffective.

Cerebral oedema—commonly appears around any sizable infarct. To prevent or reduce this a number of agents have been tried.

1. Diuretics e.g. frusemide—40–80 mg daily.
2. Mannitol—an IV infusion of 20% solution, 100–200 ml. This causes a brisk diuresis which may cause retention in elderly men. It may also cause rebound deterioration with increased oedema after the infusion has finished.
3. Glycerol—usually given for 4–7 days either orally (or by nasogastric tube), 1–2 g/kg/day in 10% solution, or IV 50 g in 500 ml of saline given over four hours. Rarely this may produce haemolysis or renal failure.
4. Dexamethasone—5 mg by injection six hourly, or 4 mg six hourly by mouth initially and then on a reducing scale. This is very effective in reducing oedema around tumours but may have little effect in acute strokes. High dose steroids may aggravate infections, provoke diabetes or even gastric haemorrhage or perforation.

Blood changes—a high PCV suggests a high viscosity and reduced cerebral blood flow. Lowering the PCV reverses these. Low molecular weight dextran (Dextran 40) may reduce plasma viscosity, blood sludging and platelet stickiness. Dextran 40 has been used in very ill stroke patients for 72 hours with some benefit but such infusions may cause circulatory overload and occasionally renal failure.

In *a 'continuing stroke'* CT scanning and CSF examination will exclude other pathology and most haemorrhages. Anticoagulant therapy here may be helpful. An IV heparin drip (continuous infusion) or bolus doses (10 000 units six hourly) can be continued for five to seven days. If the clinical situation stabilises or improves then a change to oral therapy with warfarin can be made.

In patients with a recognisable embolic source where there is a real risk of further emboli, anticoagulants may be used. A CT scan and CSF examination to exclude a haemorrhagic infarct should be performed first. These patients may need long term treatment or removal of the embolic source.

General measures: Feeding, by nasogastric tube if difficulties by mouth, skin care, regular turning and treatment of pressure areas. Bowel and bladder function needs supervision. Catheterisation may be necessary in the early stages. Physiotherapy and early mobilisation greatly helps rehabilitation and may reduce the incidence of deep vein thromboses in the legs.

About 30% of patients who have had an acute stroke are dead within one month. The mortality is higher after cerebral haemorrhage. Of the survivors about 30% are severely and permanently disabled.

Subarachnoid Haemorrhage (SAH)

This commonly presents with the acute onset of severe headache. It may be triggered by exertion or stress and in some patients the ictus may start with transient loss of consciousness, an epileptic fit or even coma. The headache may be described as a severe blow and is often accompanied by vomiting, a stiff neck, photophobia and prominent backache. In some patients there may be symptoms of focal neurological disturbance, of oculomotor upset e.g. diplopia, or even an altered mental state. Most SAHs are due to ruptured aneurysms, but they may occur from a bleeding diathesis or angioma. In the last instance, patients often have a history of fits, sometimes focal symptoms and signs and a bruit may be audible over the skull.

Patients with an SAH show signs of meningeal irritation with variable conscious levels. The last are important in management. Patients who are comatose or have a depressed conscious level do badly.

The dangers of an SAH are the high mortality and morbidity from rebleeding, although c. 15% probably die in the initial bleed. The maximum incidence of rebleeding lies in the first six weeks. For this reason suitable patients are considered for angiography (carotid and vertebral) so that if an aneurysm is demonstrated it can be clipped surgically. A few patients have multiple aneurysms. Patients with an SAH often show glycosuria and ECG changes; in part due to catecholamine release and in part due to a rise in blood pressure.

Investigation: 1. Blood tests to exclude a bleeding tendency. 2. CSF examination to confirm the diagnosis and exclude infection. 3. A CT scan may confirm the bleed and often indicate the possible site of origin (Plate 10b). 4. Plain X-rays of the skull (Plate 2b) and chest. 5. An ECG. 6. In selected patients angiography should be performed but selection is necessary so that only those patients are investigated whose age and state would indicate surgery if an accessible aneurysm was found (Plate 11a).

Treatment: Surgery has been greatly helped by the use of the dissecting microscope, reduction of cerebral oedema and controlled hypotension (e.g. by sodium nitroprusside) at operation. Timing of surgery is important weighing the risks of rebleeding in the first few days against the increased surgical mortality and morbidity at that time. Clipping of the aneurysm neck is the aim. In a few patients internal carotid artery ligation in the neck may be used in an attempt to prevent rebleeding from an aneurysm in the territory of that artery. Haematoma evacuation may be necessary. Drugs may also be used to try and prevent the break down of clot that has formed within an aneurysm. Epsilon aminocaproic acid, 18–30 g/day, or tranexamic acid, 6 g/day, have been used for this.

Patients unsuitable for surgery, usually because of their clinical state, age, or other medical causes, are treated by strict bed rest for four to six weeks. Hypertension should be controlled. One problem after an SAH is the development of arterial spasm which may cause marked clinical deterioration. At present the remedy for this is uncertain.

Transient Ischaemic Attacks (TIAs)

These are important as they may herald an acute stroke. They may occur in carotid or VB territory. Carotid territory attacks carry the worst prognosis. They are commonly due to small fibrin-platelet emboli.

Carotid territory attacks include transient amaurotic episodes—ipsilateral monocular visual loss usually described as a 'shutter closing' lasting for a minute or two. They also include symptoms of transient hemisphere upset—classically brachio-facial weakness or hemiparesis, hemisensory disturbance or if the dominant hemisphere is involved, dysphasia with speech upset. All these symptoms and signs appear contralateral to the affected carotid territory.

Vertebrobasilar territory attacks have many forms. The most common is vertigo, which may be accompanied by ataxia and dysarthria. There may be episodic visual upset—bilateral visual obscurations, teichopsia, hemianopias, diplopia or blurring. Drop attacks, falling to the ground without warning, paroxysmal headaches, and facial numbness and tingling (often circumoral) may occur. There may also be episodes of hemiparesis or hemisensory disturbance which may be difficult to distinguish from carotid territory attacks: however in VB attacks the episodes may alternate from side to side or be associated with other symptoms. Alternating hemiparetic or hemisensory attacks carry a greater stroke risk. In some patients VB attacks are precipitated by head turning.

Rare patients with VB symptoms may have a *'subclavian steal'* where a significant proximal subclavian artery stenosis or occlusion may produce reversal of blood flow away from the brain stem down one vertebral artery towards an arm. Such patients have unequal radial pulses, uneven blood pressures in the two arms and often an audible bruit at the base of the neck.

Most patients with TIAs show no abnormal signs. In a few there may be a significant bruit over a stenotic area in an extracranial feeding artery commonly the origin of the internal carotid.

Precipitating causes of TIAs and strokes are outlined in Table VI. From this it can be seen that *investigations* include a blood sample, ECG, X-rays of the chest, skull and neck. In selected patients a CT scan and angiography may be necessary.

Table VI
Precipitating Causes of Transient Ischaemic Attacks and Strokes

1. Blood	Too 'thick'	polycythaemia
	Too 'thin'	anaemia
	Inflammatory	arteritis, syphilis
	Chemistry	lipid upset, diabetes
2. Blood pressure	Too high	hypertension
	Too low	iatrogenic
3. Disorders of the heart		
(a) Rate	Too fast	supraventricular tachycardia
	Too slow	heart block
(b) Rhythm	Irregular	fibrillation
	Variable	paroxysmal changes, sick sinus
(c) Failure		falling output
4. Embolic sources		
(a) Cardiac		infarcts, valves
(b) Extracranial arteries		stenotic lesions, atheromatous ulcers
5. Mechanical compression		vertebral arteries by osteophytes

Outlook: most authors accept a stroke incidence of 30–40% following TIAs. In order to prevent strokes, assessment is made to exclude hypertension, an obvious cardiac cause, or abnormality of the blood. In particular a high PCV is associated with reduced blood flow and an increased stroke incidence.

Selected patients may be submitted to angiography, usually carotid, to try and detect atheromatous stenotic lesions (Plate 12) or ulcers in surgically accessible parts of the extracranial arteries. If such a lesion is found, disobliteration may prevent further TIAs and strokes. There is a morbidity to angiography in such arteriopaths and the best chance of finding a surgically correctable lesion lies in patients between the ages of 50–65, with a bruit, a history of carotid territory TIAs and amaurosis, a BP of > 150/90 and claudication.

In patients with significant hypertension (diastolic BP > 110) control of the BP is the first measure. In patients where no surgical lesion is demonstrated or angiography has not been performed, treatment may be by:
1. anticoagulants for six to twelve months, the time of maximal risk.
2. soluble aspirin (300–600 mg/day).

Preliminary trials suggest that low dosage aspirin (acting on platelet stickiness) reduces the incidence of TIAs and strokes. The exact dose is still uncertain.

Recently with the help of the dissecting microscope, extracranial–intracranial anastomotic operations have been carried out in a few highly selected patients with widespread disease. Here the superficial temporal artery (a branch of the external carotid) has been joined to a branch of the middle cerebral artery.

Hypertensive Encephalopathy

Such patients have a history of sudden onset headache, vomiting, often confusion, focal fits, visual upset and sometimes focal symptoms and signs. The diastolic BP is very high, often 130–140 mm Hg and needs urgent reduction.

Diazoxide (150 mg IV) is usually effective, lasting two to four hours. Hydralazine by slow IV injection (1 mg/minute to c. 10 mg) titrating the dose against the fall in BP, is an alternative. The addition of frusemide 40 mg IV reinforces these drugs and may prevent heart failure. Once the initial high

Table VII
Risk Factors Increasing the Incidence of Strokes

1. Hypertension	
2. Cardiac Causes	Embolic sources—mural infarcts, diseased valves Heart failure, Ischaemic heart disease
3. Lipid Abnormalities	particularly younger patients (< 55)
4. Diabetes mellitus	
5. Transient Ischaemic Attacks	
6. High Packed Cell Volume (PCV)	
7. Smoking	particularly males (increased risks of SAH and malignant hypertension)
8. Oral Contraceptive Pill	

BP has been lowered, standard hypotensive therapy will be necessary for long-lasting control.

Stroke Prevention

A number of risk factors are associated with a higher incidence of strokes. These are shown in Table VII.

9. EPILEPSY

Epilepsy describes patients who have repeated fits. The term should only be used when the diagnosis is established. Fits arise from a sudden excessive discharge in a local group of nerve cells or from a more widespread disturbance. Many classifications of fits have been made. A simple one (Table VIII) divides fits into those arising from (1) a generalised or centrencephalic upset or (2) those with a focal or localised origin. These overlap, for focal fits may spread and become generalised. However the important point is that focal fits suggest a site of origin in the brain where there may be a structural lesion.

Grand mal, major or tonic-clonic fits are the commonest. Some patients have a warning, they fall, stiffen, shake, and are often cyanosed. Post-ictal drowsiness, headache and confusion are common. There is often tongue biting and incontinence. Their duration is usually minutes and injuries may be sustained in such fits.

Temporal lobe epilepsy (TLE) is also common but two thirds of these patients also have major fits. The temporal lobes are areas of memory so a number of different auras may appear—memory upset, *déjà vu*, unfamiliarity, confusion, hallucinations of smell, taste, vision, and sound, anxiety or fear. Usually simple motor upsets occur with lip smacking, grimacing, swallowing, plucking at clothes or dropping objects. Many patients do not fall and the duration is brief (one to two minutes) but is usually followed by longer lasting confusion.

Table VIII
Types of Epileptic Fit

1. Generalised, centrencephalic	Grand mal, major, tonic-clonic Petit mal, absences Myoclonic myoclonic-astatic, akinetic Infantile spasms

2. Focal or partial	i. with elementary symptoms
	   motor, Jacksonian
	   sensory
	ii. with complex symptoms
	   temporal lobe (TLE)

Focal fits may be *motor or sensory*. Motor attacks arise in the motor cortex starting with involuntary movements in the thumb, big toe or corner of the mouth. The movements may spread in a hemiparetic distribution or become generalised. Consciousness may not be lost and post-ictally there may be transient focal signs. Sensory attacks usually consist of tingling, numbness, 'shocks' or even painful sensations spreading into one half of the body, face and limbs. They may be hard to differentiate from sensory TIAs. These focal attacks usually have an underlying local structural cause.

Petit mal is commonly misdiagnosed. It occurs largely in children between the ages of 5 and 15. It is rare to start before the age of two or in adult life. Attacks or 'absences' consist of brief loss of awareness lasting 5–15 seconds when children are out of touch with their surrounds. Recovery often occurs with visible blinking and there is no falling. Sometimes attacks occur in series. Although most patients with petit mal find their attacks cease in adult life, a significant proportion develop major fits.

Minor fits describe a number of different types of episodes usually with transient loss of awareness or consciousness. They include *myoclonic jerks* or starts. these may occur in isolation, herald a more major fit or be seen in patients with anoxic brain damage, uraemia or in rare degenerative brain diseases (page 108). *Akinetic attacks* describe episodes with sudden falling without warning and with no convulsing. Many of these patients have other types of fits.

Fits in Children

Febrile convulsions are common in children (some 3–5%) and occur with a rise in temperature. The problem is that a proportion of these children (10–15%) go on to develop epileptic fits and there is evidence to suggest a prolonged febrile convulsion may cause anoxic brain damage in the temporal lobe making this a site of origin for future temporal lobe fits.

Certain features predispose children to continuing attacks: a positive family history, a prolonged fit (> 30 minutes), repeated attacks, a focal fit, persisting neurological signs after a fit and an early age of onset (< 18 months). In patients with these adverse risk factors, prophylactic anticonvulsant treatment is advised, probably using valproate or phenobarbitone.

It should be emphasised that in very young children *meningitis* may present with a fit and there may be no meningism.

In *neonates* tonic fits may occur, often from brain damage. Clonic fits may also occur, sometimes focal, and these may have metabolic (e.g. hypoglycaemia) or structural causes (Table IX).

Infantile spasms (hypsarrhythmia, salaam attacks, West's syndrome) describe a type of epilepsy occurring in infants. The attacks start between the

Table IX
Causes of Epileptic Fits

Adults	
Idiopathic, cryptogenic	Commonest, often start in 'teens
Trauma	Penetrating head injuries-high incidence; birth
Infective	Meningitis, encephalitis, abscess
Vascular	Infarcts, hypertensive encephalopathy, aneurysms, angiomata
Tumours	Primary—benign or malignant, metastases
Metabolic	Low sugar, calcium, sodium; uraemia, hepatic failure, porphyria
Drugs	Withdrawal—alcohol, barbiturates. Isoniazid, tricyclic antidepressants
Poisons	Lead
Degenerative	Alzheimer
Neonates	
First three days of life	Cerebral damage — Haemorrhage / Anoxia
	Hypoglycaemia, (hypocalcaemia)
Days 7–10	Metabolic—low sugar, calcium, magnesium, pyridoxine deficiency, rare inborn errors of metabolism
All Ages	Meningitis
	Trauma
	Tumours (rare)
	Phakomatoses e.g. tuberose sclerosis

ages of three to nine months. In a typical attack, babies flex the body from the waist in a salaam drawing up their legs. Many of the infants have evidence of early brain damage and in many children there is a poor prognosis with a high incidence of mental retardation.

Investigations

The most important of these is an account of an attack by an eye-witness. In most adults an FBC, ESR, X-rays of the skull and chest, and an EEG are valuable. Many other tests may be necessary particularly if there is diagnostic doubt (Table IX). These may include a fasting blood glucose, or one taken in an attack, calcium, WR and ECG and testing the urine for porphyrins.

If there is a suggestion of a focal onset, persisting abnormal signs, or those of raised ICP, then a CT scan should be performed. In particular this will show a tumour. A radio-isotope scan may be useful if CT scans are not available. The CSF may need examination if infection is suspected, particularly in infants.

Most adults have no abnormal signs and routine investigations prove normal. The EEG may be abnormal. However in 'normal adults' some 10–15% may show EEG abnormalities so the presence of an abnormality is not diagnostic of epilepsy and a 'normal' EEG does not exclude the diagnosis.

A local 'spike' focus may suggest a focal site of origin and a slow wave focus may suggest an underlying structural fault such as a tumour (in only 15% of patients with late onset epilepsy is a tumour the cause). Repetitive generalised three per second spike and wave discharges on the EEG may be diagnostic of petit mal if accompanied by clinical features. A rather atypical similar pattern may occur with other types of fits.

In neonates metabolic screening is essential; this should include an urinary amino acid chromatogram and screening for sugars.

Treatment

Metabolic causes may be remedied with cessation of fits. However in about 80% of epileptic patients anticonvulsants will control but not cure the fits. Wherever possible one drug alone should be used. The dose should be increased until there is good control or the appearance of toxic side-effects. Control has been greatly aided by the use of anticonvulsant blood levels. It should be emphasised that many drugs e.g. phenytoin or phenobarbitone, have a long half life (days) so that they need to be given regularly for 7–10 days before a steady plasma level is reached. Most anticonvulsants can be given twice daily which aids compliance. Table X suggests the drugs

Table X
Anticonvulsant Levels

Drug	Usual adult dose mg/day	Half-life (hours)	Days to reach plateau	Therapeutic level µg/ml	Therapeutic level µmol/l
Carbamazepine (Tegretol)	800–1000	8–46	2–3	4–10	17–42
Ethosuximide (Zarontin)	750	30 (children)	7	40–120	280–840
		60–100 (adults)	7		
Phenobarbitone (Luminal)	90–180	36–72 (children)	7+	15–40	66–176
		48–140 (adults)	7+		
Primidone* (Mysoline)	750	3–12	7+	5–15	23–69
Phenytoin** (Epanutin)	200–400	22 ± 9	7–10	10–20	40–80
Valproate (Epilim)	600–2000	8–15	1–3	60–100	420–700***

* the majority is broken down to phenobarbitone
**varies with the dose
***variation between different reports

available, their half life, adult dose range and therapeutic levels. Table XI suggests drugs of choice to start treatment. In a few patients polypharmacy appears necessary to achieve control and some patients may be receiving two or even three separate drugs.

Table XI
Drugs used in the Control of Epileptic Fits

Seizure type	Anticonvulsant Drug
Grand mal	Phenytoin, carbamazepine, phenobarbitone, primidone, valproate
Focal	Phenytoin, carbamazepine, primidone
Temporal lobe	Carbamazepine, phenytoin, primidone
Petit mal	Valproate, ethosuximide
Myoclonic, akinetic	Valproate, clonazepam, nitrazepam
Infantile spasms	ACTH, clonazepam, nitrazepam
Febrile convulsions	Valproate, phenobarbitone (for prevention)
Serial fits	Intravenous clonazepam, diazepam, phenytoin Intramuscular paraldehyde
Status epilepticus	Intravenous clonazepam, diazepam, thiopentone, chlormethiazole

Side effects

All anticonvulsants have side-effects. Some are 'allergic', e.g. skin rashes or gastro-intestinal upset, some due to dose-related toxicity—particularly drowsiness, ataxia, nystagmus and dysarthria, and some appear specific, e.g. on the bone marrow. Reports of osteomalacia have appeared in a few patients receiving treatment for many years.

Phenobarbitone causes drowsiness, irritability and behaviour disturbances in children, depression in adolescents and confusion in the elderly. Phenytoin is likely to cause intoxication in high dosage. Hirsutism, gum hypertrophy, marrow depression and lymph gland hyperplasia have all been reported. Carbamazepine in addition to intoxication, may rarely cause marrow depression with aplastic anaemia and also liver upset. Primidone is broken down into phenobarbitone and phenylethylmalonamide so phenobarbitone and primidone should not be prescribed together. Its side-effects are similar to phenobarbitone but it may cause an acute toxic reaction on starting treatment with nausea, vomiting, prostration and cerebellar signs. To avoid this it should be introduced slowly.

Valproate is well tolerated and effective in the control of both petit mal and major fits. It has a low incidence of side-effects but gastric irritation, hair thinning, liver damage and thrombocytopenia have been reported. Benzodiazepines include clonazepam and nitrazepam. Side-effects of these are largely drowsiness, increased secretions and in high doses ataxia. Oral diazepam is not an anti-convulsant.

Other Causes of Transient Loss of Consciousness

Many patients present with a history of 'blackouts' or transient loss of consciousness. Although a proportion may be due to epileptic fits many are not. In the elderly vascular causes are common.

Syncope, faints: a fall in cerebral blood flow usually produces warning symptoms; loss of consciousness is brief without sequelae. There may be clear provoking factors e.g. standing in a hot room, after an injection. There is an overlap with fits as these may be triggered by prolonged anoxia, as in patients who have fainted and are supported in a chair or held upright.

Cardiac causes: a changing heart rate or rhythm, paroxysmal tachycardia, heart block or 'sick sinus' may cause a fall in cerebral perfusion. Exercise in patients with tight aortic stenosis may also cause loss of consciousness. ECG records or an ambulatory 24 hour ECG tape recording may aid diagnosis. A postural fall in blood pressure may occur, especially in elderly patients on hypotensive treatment, and in diabetics with an autonomic neuropathy. TIAs in VB territory may cause drop attacks.

Cough syncope may follow prolonged coughing and *micturition syncope* affects men standing to empty their bladders, often at night. *Carotid sinus sensitivity* may cause loss of consciousness. Here stimulation of the carotid sinus in the neck may cause reflex slowing of the heart rate and in sensitive patients atrial asystole.

Migraine affecting the hind-brain circulation may cause loss of consciousness. Usually young women present with attacks of intense occipital headache, severe enough to make them lie down. There then may be loss of consciousness for 20–30 minutes. There are often other symptoms of brain stem disturbance.

Patients with an intermittent *obstructive hydrocephalus*, e.g. a colloid cyst of the third ventricle, may develop attacks of crescendo headache. At the height of the pain there may be collapse with loss of consciousness. Many patients show disc swelling and some dementia. A CT scan will confirm the diagnosis.

In some *head injuries* there may be brief loss of consciousness with amnesia which may extend to cover the time of the accident so that details cannot be remembered. Middle aged women may develop drop attacks, falling forward without warning, often while walking, sometimes sustaining injuries. These have been described as *benign cryptogenic drop attacks* (Stevens & Matthews, 1973). Investigations prove normal and the attacks are not influenced by anticonvulsants. Their mechanism is uncertain.

Metabolic causes are rare but include *hypoglycaemia*, most commonly from insulin overdosage in diabetics but very rarely from an insulinoma. Patients may show disturbed behaviour, seem drunk with slurred speech, unsteadiness and appear pale and sweating before consciousness is lost. A blood sample in an attack confirms the diagnosis and the response to IV dextrose is rapid. Occasionally hypoglycaemia may present with focal neurological signs.

Hyperventilation, more common in young women, will cause a respiratory alkalosis with tingling in the extremities and around the mouth. If this continues carpo-pedal spasm, muscular twitching and even loss of consciousness may follow. A trial with overbreathing may produce identical symptoms.

Hypocalcaemia can provoke true fits. It may also cause tetany with carpo-pedal spasm, muscle stiffness, cramps, and tingling in the extremities and around the mouth. Patients may also develop cataracts and disc swelling. A low serum calcium confirms the diagnosis.

Transient global amnesia usually arises on a vascular basis, occurring in older patients producing total amnesia often for a few hours. Personal identity is usually retained but patients appear confused, repeatedly asking what they are doing or where they are. Similar but much briefer lasting amnesia may follow TLE.

Narcolepsy is a sleep disorder where patients have disturbed night time sleep and brief spells in the day of an overwhelming desire to sleep. They are easily aroused from these episodes. A proportion may also have sleep paralysis, hypnagogic hallucinations and cataplexy. In the last sudden emotional upset, e.g. laughter or anger, may cause loss of muscle tone with falling. Many of these symptoms are helped by treatment with imipramine or clomipramine. Actual narcoleptic episodes may be helped with amphetamines: these are habit-forming drugs. Methylphenidate (10 mg b.d. or t.i.d.) is most commonly used.

Hysterical fits may appear causing diagnostic difficulty, particularly as they may occur in patients who also have true epileptic fits. Often attacks have an audience, bizarre postures may appear and struggling seems proportional to the degree of restraint. Tongue biting and incontinence do not occur. During an episode the eye lids may be hard to open, the corneal and oculo-vestibular reflexes are spared and the plantar responses remain flexor. In most instances in-patient observation is the best method of determining the mechanism if there is doubt. This may be aided by video recording with simultaneous EEG telemetry. It has been suggested that true major fits are followed by a rise in the serum prolactin which does not occur in spurious attacks (Trimble, 1978).

In children aged between six months and five years, *breath holding attacks* may occur. Usually frustrated or frightened children who are crying may stop breathing. Such children collapse and appear pale and limp. In these children ocular compression may produce asystole. In a second type of attack, children may stop breathing and become cyanosed. They are limp initially but then may show some clonic jerks. These attacks may be frequent and frightening but appear self-limiting and the EEG is usually normal.

Children may also develop *benign paroxysmal vertigo*. Older children will describe giddiness but younger ones may just stop playing, go pale, and hold on for support. They may cry or even vomit. The attacks are of short duration (minutes) and commonly occur between the ages of three and eight years. If caloric tests are performed, there is often a canal paresis. With time these attacks cease.

10. HEADACHE

Headache is the commonest symptom of patients seen in neurological clinics. It is helpful to determine (i) the duration, (ii) the frequency, (iii) the mode of onset or precipitants, (iv) the site and quality of the pain, and (v) the aggravating or relieving features.

Acute severe headache of sudden onset suggests a vascular or infective cause, less commonly a sudden rise in ICP. The common vascular causes of headache are migraine, haemorrhage (SAH or intracerebral) and less commonly from thrombo-embolic infarction or an arteritis.

Migraine

This usually causes acute attacks of severe headache, often hemicranial but sometimes generalised. The pain increases in intensity to a severe throbbing which may be accompanied by nausea, vomiting, photophobia and prostration. The attacks often last between several hours to one to two days. In many patients early in an attack, often before the onset of severe headache, there may be transient visual symptoms (flashing lights, colours, patches of visual loss or blurring) and less commonly transient hemisensory, hemiparetic or speech upsets. These often last 10–30 minutes, occasionally longer. Basilar territory migraine may occur with transient hind-brain ischaemic symptoms and rarely loss of consciousness. Even more rare are attacks of ophthalmoplegic migraine where an oculomotor palsy may appear in an attack. The palsy may persist for days or even weeks.

Migraine is more common in women. There is often a positive family history and an association with travel sickness. Many triggers are recognised—alcohol, certain food substances (e.g chocolate, cheese), stress, hormonal changes (the contraceptive pill), bright light, head injuries, hypoglycaemia. Very rarely migraine attacks may be symptomatic of an underlying angioma or vascular cerebral tumour.

Treatment: (i) Precipitants should be avoided. (ii) In an *acute attack* appropriate simple analgesics should be given. Soluble aspirin 600–900 mg given at the onset is often effective in adults. Troublesome nausea may be relieved by metoclopramide 10 mg. If nausea and vomiting are severe, oral drugs may be ineffective; a Cafergot suppository or one of prochlorperazine 25 mg rectally may be useful. Alternatively an injection of codeine phosphate 30–60 mg IM may be used. In acute attacks oral ergotamine may be useful, taken as early as possible, although some patients are upset by this. Care must be taken to avoid excess doses of ergotamine with the development of habituation and the appearance of withdrawal headache. (iii) In about two thirds of patients, frequent severe attacks of migraine can be reduced by the regular intake of certain drugs. These include Bellergal (a mixture of belladonna alkaloids, ergotamine and phenobarbitone), promethazine, prochlorperazine, clonidine, pizotifen, propranolol, and methysergide. The last should only be used in short courses (less than twelve weeks) as there is a risk of retroperitoneal fibrosis with prolonged use.

Migrainous neuralgia (cluster headache, sphenopalatine or vidian neuralgia)—commonly affects men with recurring episodes of intense pain centred in and around one eye usually lasting 45–90 minutes. The attacks of pain tend to recur on successive nights over several weeks awakening patients. They may also occur in the day. At the height of the pain there may be vasomotor features with ptosis, conjunctival suffusion, lachrymation, pupillary miosis and nasal stuffiness on the affected side.

Treatment: most attacks respond to ergotamine. This can be given by suppository (Cafergot) one nocte, for five successive nights omitting the dose on the sixth to see if the bout has ended. Oral ergotamine is often ineffective but lithium has been used. Surgical destructive lesions may be made in the trigeminal or sphenopalatine ganglion if medical measures fail.

Other Causes of Headache

Subarachnoid haemorrhage may present with headache of explosive onset (page 58). Acute headache may also occur with meningitis, with intracranial infections (page 44) or local sinus infections. With sinusitis there is usually local tenderness, sometimes swelling, and often nasal congestion with purulent catarrh. Dental sepsis may cause facial pain sometimes with spread to the head. Acute inflammatory eye disorders and acute glaucoma may cause acute headache. In the last, the eye is usually suffused, locally tender and there is visual disturbance.

Raised intracranial pressure may produce headache, often worse on waking, easing within one to two hours. Commonly such headaches have recurred irregularly over a few weeks. The pain may be throbbing or bursting and is aggravated by any manoeuvres that raise ICP e.g. coughing, laughing, sneezing, bending, bowel opening, intercourse and exertion. The pain, which may be relieved by simple analgesics, is often accompanied by nausea and vomiting. Very commonly other symptoms are present as drowsiness, confusion, behaviour change, fits, focal disturbances, unsteadiness etc. Posterior fossa masses causing elevated ICP may produce pain at the back of the head with neck stiffness. If the elevated ICP has caused severe papilloedema then an ominous symptom may be *transient visual obscurations*, triggered by bending, exertion etc.

Cranial arteritis, temporal or giant cell arteritis, occurs in patients over the age of 60, commonly affecting the superficial temporal arteries where the vessel may be acutely tender or thickened. The danger lies in thrombotic occlusion of the affected vessel. If this is in the retina or optic nerve, sudden irreversible blindness may occur. Patients usually feel unwell with severe headache and local scalp tenderness. They may complain of joint pains, malaise, night sweats and a low grade fever. Tenderness of affected vessels is usually present and biopsy of such will confirm the diagnosis. However the ESR is high, usually > 60 mm/hour, and if the diagnosis is clinically suspect and the ESR high patients should start immediate treatment with high doses of steroids—prednisolone 60 mg/day, which should produce rapid relief of symptoms. The dose may later be slowly reduced, monitoring progress clinically and with the ESR. Often patients require a low maintenance dose of 10–15 mg/day for six to twelve months. There is also an association with polymyalgia rheumatica.

Post lumbar puncture headache occurs as patients are mobilised and is a low pressure headache giving symptoms when patients are erect, easing on lying. It is probably caused by a CSF leak from the puncture site and may take some days to settle. Sometimes there is also pain in the neck and back and even neck stiffness. These may raise fears of iatrogenic meningitis but no fever should be present. Bed rest lying flat, or with the foot of the bed elevated may hasten recovery. Fluids should be encouraged. Lying prone for the first few hours after the lumbar puncture may reduce the incidence.

Trigeminal neuralgia

This affects older patients. It consists of intense stabs of pain in usually the distribution of the maxillary or mandibular divisions of the trigeminal nerve, on one side. The pain may be triggered by contact, movement or even cold and is severe enough to make patients cry out, stop eating or washing their faces. It seldom occurs in sleep. Often there are spontaneous remissions lasting months or years. Rarely the glossopharyngeal nerve may be affected. In younger patients it may be symptomatic of multiple sclerosis (MS).

Treatment: most patients respond to carbamazepine. In the elderly the dose may need to be increased slowly as ataxia is the main dose-limiting side-effect. Often doses of 600–800 mg/day are necessary to control a severe episode. When this has subsided the drug can be slowly tapered off. Other drugs have been used, including phenytoin and clonazepam. In a small number of patients trigeminal root section or ganglion injection with alcohol may be necessary to control the pain. Such destructive measures may leave the face numb.

Trauma

A head injury may produce a *subdural haematoma*. This may occur acutely within hours or days of injury causing a deteriorating conscious level with the appearance of focal signs (page 131). More commonly a chronic subdural haematoma may appear, particularly in the elderly, and in about half of these patients there may be no history of head injury. Patients complain of headache varying in severity which may be accompanied by a fluctuating conscious level and mental changes—often confusion or dementia. In most patients focal signs may be present, although again these may vary, and even appear on the same side as the clot. In some patients there are bilateral haematomata. As the ICP rises, tentorial herniation starts and there is loss of upgaze with mild ptosis. Later there may be pupillary inequality and a third nerve lesion. Some patients show papilloedema.

Plain skull X-rays may show displacement of a calcified pineal but diagnosis is best made with a CT scan (Plate 9a). Occasionally the haematomata may appear isodense so that shifts are important. Treatment is by surgical evacuation and burr holes should be made bilaterally, unless a haematoma is of minimal size causing no shift of mid-line structures.

Chronic headache

This is all too common. In many patients with recurring severe episodes, migraine is the cause.

'Tension' headache may be the cause of constant daily headache present over many years or months. The pain is often described as a 'band, weight, or pressure' throughout the waking hours, fluctuating in severity and often worse at the end of the day. Superimposed stabs of severe pain may occur. Many patients with such headache may also be *depressed*. If so the headache may follow the pattern of their depression with early waking, and pain appearing shortly after this.

Tension headaches may be relieved by strong reassurance coupled with an anxiolytic. The benzodiazepines, e.g. diazepam, which have muscle relaxant properties may be helpful. Many other preparations are used—some combine simple analgesics with a relaxant or tranquilliser. If significant depression is a feature then an anti-depressant, often given as a single dose at bed-time, may be effective.

Investigations: in most patients the history, examination findings and presumed diagnosis will indicate the necessary investigations.

An FBC, ESR, and X-rays of the skull and chest should be performed. The need for CSF examination, a CT scan or other procedures as temporal artery biopsy will depend on the circumstances.

11. GIDDINESS

Giddiness or dizziness is a common symptom and because it is so subjective it is important to analyse what patients mean by this. It is necessary to check if the symptom arises in patients' heads and to define whether there is vertigo, an hallucination of movement (usually a feeling of rotation or falling), whether there is unsteadiness (imbalance) or whether there is faintness or light-headedness.

Vertigo

Vertigo commonly occurs in attacks of variable duration. It is helpful to know if these recur, for how long, any precipitating factors, the mode of onset, any associated features and any measures that afford relief. In many attacks of acute vertigo there are complaints of nausea, vomiting, prostration and feelings of fear—all features found in bouts of acute *motion sickness*.

Vertigo may arise from a number of sites (Table XII). Labyrinthine lesions may cause acute distress. Common causes of acute paroxysmal vertigo include:

1. *Benign positional vertigo*—patients complain of acute vertigo triggered by a sudden change of position e.g. lying down, sitting up or turning. There are no abnormal signs except that positional testing (page 11) will produce rotatory nystagmus after a latent period accompanied by vertigo. If the test is repeated it fatigues and the lesion appears to lie in the lower otolith under test. In some patients there is a history of preceding trauma or a respiratory infection. The condition appears self-limiting and with time most patients improve. Vestibular sedatives, as cinnarizine or prochlorperazine, may also give relief.

2. *Vestibular neuronitis*—patients present with acute vertigo lasting several days. Initially this is severe, aggravated by movement, and accompanied by prostration, nausea and vomiting. There may also be unsteadiness. No cochlear signs or symptoms appear but there may be spontaneous nystagmus with abnormal caloric tests initially. Over some weeks improvement occurs although there may be paroxysmal vertigo triggered by movement for a time. The cause is thought viral and treatment is by rest, parenteral anti-emetics and vestibular sedatives.

3. *Menière's disease*—occurs in older patients causing acute attacks of vertigo accompanied by vomiting and prostration, usually lasting 15–90 minutes. However many patients may feel unwell for some hours. Most attacks are preceded by a sensation of fullness in the head and with tinnitus. Between attacks examination commonly shows deafness which is perceptive, with loudness recruitment and tone decay (indicating a cochlear lesion). Caloric tests will show a canal paresis, a directional preponderance or a combination of the two. During an attack nystagmus may be seen and patients are unsteady. With time some patients develop bilateral disease. The cause is thought to be due to a distension of the endolymph system. Various treatments are used: they include salt restriction with the addition of diuretics, vestibular sedatives and even surgical destruction of the affected labyrinth.

In the brain stem acute vertigo may be caused by attacks of *migraine*, or transient *basilar ischaemia.* Other vascular conditions which cause a drop in cerebral perfusion may also be involved e.g. postural hypotension, or changes in heart rate or rhythm. Longer lasting symptoms may occur with *infarcts.* Here vertigo is usually associated with ataxia, vomiting, hiccup and often symptoms referable to damage to the lower cranial nerve nuclei and the long tracts passing through the brain stem (page 55).

Plaques of *demyelination* within the brain stem may cause episodes of

Table XII
Causes of Vertigo

Peripheral Labyrinthine Lesions	
Acute infections	Suppurative otitis media, cholesteatoma, zoster
Benign positional vertigo	
Vestibular neuronitis	
Menière's disease	
Vestibular Nerve	
Acoustic neuroma	Rare episodic
Drugs	Streptomycin, gentamicin
Brain Stem	
Vascular	Migraine,
	Infarct, haemorrhage,
	Basilar ischaemia,
	Perfusion upsets—BP fall,
	Changes in heart rate or rhythm
Inflammatory	Multiple sclerosis
Tumours	Acoustic neuroma, posterior fossa masses (more ataxia)
Metabolic	Wernicke's encephalopathy
Drugs	Alcohol, phenytoin, barbiturates (also central)
Central	
Epilepsy	TLE
Tumours	Raised ICP, large masses with displacement or Hydrocephalus
Psychogenic	Hyperventilation, anxiety

more prolonged upset with vomiting, vertigo and ataxia. These are usually younger patients. There may be ocular signs, nystagmus and an internuclear ophthalmoplegia, and facial sensory loss and weakness. Limb and cerebellar signs may also be present. A past history of neurological disturbance, abnormal VERs or auditory evoked potentials, and an abnormal CSF may support the diagnosis.

Wernicke's encephalopathy, a rare condition which may be missed, may present with vertigo and ocular symptoms (page 122). Giddiness may also occur as the aura in many types of *epileptic fit*. Vertigo may be produced by *drugs and alcohol*. In acute alcoholic poisoning vertigo is common. Some drugs damage the eighth nerve e.g. streptomycin, gentamicin, others cause ataxia such as phenytoin, carbamazepine, barbiturates and benzodiazepines.

Imbalance

Chronic unsteadiness or imbalance is very common in the elderly. Here it is likely that a number of causes summate—neuronal degeneration in cerebellar and basal ganglia pathways (causing ataxia of stance and gait with impaired balance and disordered righting reflexes), often aggravated by variable cerebral perfusion and vascular damage.

In a few patients rare *degenerative disorders* of cerebellar pathways may be responsible. In younger patients, a spino-cerebellar degeneration as Friedreich's ataxia may present (page 102). Myxoedema may rarely cause cerebellar disturbance. Patients here may show delayed relaxation of the ankle jerks. *Tumours* in the posterior fossa (more common in children) may present with unsteadiness. An acoustic neuroma may produce progressive ataxia with symptoms of eighth and fifth nerve involvement (page 83). In older patients metastases are relatively common in the posterior fossa. Occasionally an obstructive hydrocephalus may present with unsteadiness, sometimes with an accompanying dementia. Very large supratentorial tumours, causing considerable displacements, may present with symptoms of dizziness and unsteadiness.

Sensory ataxia from loss of joint position sense may also cause ataxia. Here marked Rombergism and appropriate sensory loss with absent ankle jerks are common, although such disorders are rare, e.g. tabes dorsalis.

In many patients vague symptoms of light-headedness, imbalance or giddiness may be prominent. Some of these patients show no abnormal signs and their circulatory system appears stable. Eighth nerve function is normal (caloric tests and audiometry). *Psychogenic causes* may be responsible and are seen in some anxious patients. Hyperventilation sometimes is a cause.

Investigations

In all patients examination should be accompanied by further tests of the eighth nerve system, including audiometry, caloric and positional tests. Electronystagmography may add much further detail (page 25). In addition routine blood tests, an ECG, an EEG (if indicated) and X-rays of the chest, skull and internal auditory canals may be carried out. In further selected patients a CT scan and CSF examination may be necessary.

12. TUMOURS

Because of a selected population, cerebral tumours appear common in a neurological unit. A number of classifications of tumours are used and a simple one is given in Table XIII. The incidence of different types of tumour varies widely; in a neurosurgical series the incidence of metastases was 4–8% but in a pathological series c. 20%. Many tumours are benign and may be totally resectable offering a good chance of 'cure'. With modern surgical techniques e.g. the operating microscope, and better neuro-anaesthesia, mortality and morbidity have been reduced. In children tumours are particularly liable to arise in the posterior fossa. It should be emphasised that other mass lesions e.g. cerebral abscesses or subdural haematomata, may present like tumours.

Tumours present in many ways. These include features of:
1. Elevated intracranial pressure (ICP)
2. Focal neurological signs
3. Epileptic fits
4. Hydrocephalus
5. Endocrine disturbances

There may also be false localising signs caused by compression of structures remote from the tumour.

Table XIII
Cerebral Tumours

	Incidence	Type
Adults		
Benign	Meningioma	13–19%
	Pituitary	8–18%
	Acoustic neuroma	6–9%
	Angioma	5%
	Cysts	
Malignant		
Primary	Glioma	43–48%
Secondary	Metastatic	5–20%*
Children		
Posterior Fossa		
	Medulloblastoma	21%
	Cerebellar astrocytoma	17%
	Ependymoma	6%
	Pontine glioma	
Supratentorial		
	Craniopharyngioma	
	Ependymoma	

*these incidence figures are from neurosurgical series; in a general hospital metastases have a higher incidence

Elevated ICP

Classically the symptoms and signs are headache (page 71), vomiting and visual upset. Vomiting is commonly associated with the headache but lesions around the fourth ventricle may cause this on its own. As the ICP rises it may cause pressure on the optic nerves producing papilloedema. Unlike patients with optic neuritis, many with papilloedema have no change in their visual acuity. With chronic papilloedema there may be failing vision with enlarging blind spots and constricting visual fields. If the ICP is very high transient amaurosis may occur with loss of vision lasting for a few seconds, provoked by manoeuvres which further raise the pressure e.g. bending, coughing, exercise. This is a danger symptom. However a significant number of patients with elevated ICP show no papilloedema.

Visual upset may occur with the development of diplopia—commonly a single or bilateral abducens palsy often produced by high pressure alone (a false localising sign). In mild degree, the patient may complain of visual blurring.

Most patients with elevated ICP also show *mental changes* or *clouding of consciousness*; these features may be more apparent to relatives. Many patients appear drowsy, later becoming confused, apathetic and less accessible: some show personality change or even frank dementia.

Pressure Cones: the skull is a rigid container so that increasing ICP may cause displacement of the contents in the various compartments. This is a pressure cone and can occur at two important sites: (i) through the tentorial hiatus, where a supratentorial mass causes downward herniation of the uncus and hippocampal gyrus which are caught on the free edge of the tent; (ii) through the foramen magnum, where the cerebellar tonsils herniate downwards compressing the medulla.

A *transtentorial cone* causes a progressive deteriorating conscious level often with initial fluctuations, accompanied by signs of an ipsilateral oculomotor palsy. This causes pupillary dilatation and loss of pupil reactions. Later a complete ophthalmoplegia appears. Displacement of the lower part of the temporal lobe medially may compress the internal capsule producing a contralateral hemiparesis, then decorticate and later decerebrate postures. Rarely there may be compression of the posterior cerebral artery with the appearance of a hemianopia. These cone signs may become bilateral with fixed dilated pupils, extensor rigidity, a slowed pulse and irregular respiration. By this stage cerebral damage may be irreversible.

A *foramen magnum cone* again causes a deteriorating conscious level, sometimes with the appearance of a 'trance-like' state. There is usually neck stiffness and disordered respiration, often with irregular periods of increasing apnoea. The pulse slows, the blood pressure rises and there may be sudden death.

The recognition of such pressure cones indicates the need for *urgent* measures to reduce ICP and establish a definitive diagnosis.

Focal symptoms and signs and epileptic fits

These usually reflect neuronal irritation or destruction and vary with the site of involvement.

Frontal lobe: lesions may be silent particularly in the non-dominant hemisphere. Many patients show changes in intellectual function, personality and behaviour. These may be accompanied by apathy, fatigue and dulled emotions. Posteriorly placed lesions may produce a contralateral hemiparesis and in the dominant hemisphere a non-fluent dysphasia (Broca's type) with telegrammatic speech. Lesions on the orbital surface of the frontal lobe may cause anosmia and in the paracentral lobule urinary incontinence. Some patients may show a grasp reflex and even tremor and extra-pyramidal signs. Focal fits may occur often with turning of the head and eyes away from the affected frontal lobe. These fits may become generalised.

Parietal lobe: anteriorly placed lesions cause a contralateral hemiparesis. As the lesion extends further back contralateral hemisensory upsets occur. These commonly affect discriminative functions so that there is impairment of two point appreciation, graphaesthesiae, stereognosis, joint position and tactile localisation. There may also be sensory inattention which may be visual. In some patients a contralateral hemianopia may occur. If the dominant hemisphere is involved there is often dysphasia, with problems in reading, writing and calculation. In some patients with parietal lesions there may be neglect or loss of awareness (agnosia) of the affected side. Such agnosias may include denial of impaired function. An apraxia, where there is loss of performance although no motor deficit or gross sensory loss, may appear. Patients with non-dominant parietal lesions may show perceptual difficulties (e.g. in picture recognition) and visuo-spatial upsets (e.g. difficulty in constructional tasks).

Fits with a focal signature, either motor or sensory, are common in parietal lesions.

Temporal lobe: lesions in the non-dominant side may be silent until they have reached a large size. It should be emphasised that the dominant hemisphere is the left in right handed subjects and also in c. 70% of sinistrals. Dominant temporal lobe lesions are likely to cause dysphasia, nominal and expressive. TLE is very common in patients with tumours at this site. Often such attacks are heralded by an aura. This may be olfactory, gustatory, or linked with memory (page 62). Many such patients may also show irritability with aggressive outbursts and emotional instability.

Lesions deep in the medial part of the temporal lobe cause severe memory loss, particularly for recently acquired material, although this is most marked in patients with bilateral lesions.

Visual field defects are common with temporal lobe lesions. They may start as an upper quadrantanopia and spread to a hemianopia.

Occipital lobe: lesions here commonly cause a contralateral field defect, usually a hemianopia (Fig. 1, page 7). Fits are less common but may have visual hallucinations as an aura.

Posterior fossa: tumours in adults may arise in the cerebellar hemispheres causing lateralised inco-ordination and clumsiness in the ipsilateral limbs. If the lesion lies in the midline, truncal ataxia, affecting stance and gait, may be prominent. These signs are often associated with dysarthria, coarse nystagmus (to the side of the lesion) and an intention tremor.

Lesions arising in the brain stem will affect the cranial nerve nuclei on the same side at that level and the long tracts passing through that region which supply the limbs. Intrinsic pontine tumours may be very slow-growing causing progressive deficit over a long period without features of elevated ICP. Most posterior fossa tumours produce an obstructive hydrocephalus with features of elevated ICP.

Hydrocephalus

This may be caused by cerebral tumours obstructing the CSF pathways leading to progressive ventricular enlargement. This is commonly associated with mental changes and dementia which may be so severe that they prevent patients complaining. Many such patients are also unsteady (another false localising sign) and have signs of elevated ICP (e.g. papilloedema). If the enlarging third ventricle compresses the upper mid-brain there may be loss of upgaze, and later impaired ocular convergence, ptosis and even pupillary light-near dissociation. Urinary incontinence, with lost awareness for this, may also occur. Occasionally the obstructive hydrocephalus may be intermittent, e.g. a colloid cyst of the third ventricle obstructing the foramen of Monro: here there may be attacks of crescendo headache with loss of consciousness.

Endocrine and hypothalamic symptoms

These may be produced by pituitary tumours or those extending into the hypothalamus. Most pituitary tumours are non-secreting chromophobe adenomata and produce symptoms of hypopituitarism. These may be accompanied by headache and visual symptoms. In females menstrual disturbances and infertility are the earliest endocrine features, in males loss of libido. Later features of depressed thyroid function appear often with a typical appearance of pale smooth skin, thinning hair, and in males reduced shaving. Later adrenal function may be depressed with little reserve for acute upsets.

Some pituitary tumours show excess hormonal secretions, as growth hormone in acromegaly, leading to the characteristic appearance with overgrowth of the face, hands and feet. There is often headache, excess sweating, diabetes, a proximal myopathy and entrapment neuropathies. Other actively secreting tumours produce ACTH with features of Cushing's syndrome—obesity, rounding of the face, a 'buffalo hump', striae, hypertension, osteoporosis and hirsutism. Recently prolactin-secreting tumours have been increasingly found. They cause infertility with amenorrhoea and galactorrhoea in women, and loss of libido and impotence in men. All secreting tumours as they enlarge may produce headache and visual symptoms.

Tumours arising in or extending into the posterior pituitary and hypothalamus may cause diabetes insipidus with polyuria and polydipsia, obesity and hypersomnia. Later they may produce an obstructive hydrocephalus.

Childhood Cerebral Tumours

The common cerebral tumours in adults and children are given in Table XIII. In children most tumours arise in the posterior fossa and c. 50% are 'benign'. In children younger than 13, the commonest symptoms of intracranial tumours were vomiting 61%, headache 49%, ataxia 42%, impaired consciousness 37%, squint 19% and fits 11% (Till, 1975). About 50% of children with cerebral tumours have papilloedema.

The commonest childhood tumours are *medulloblastomas*. These often arise in the roof of the fourth ventricle and may seed along the neuraxis producing deposits in the spinal cord: some are supratentorial. Tumour cells may be found in the CSF. They are highly malignant and present with features of elevated ICP, particularly vomiting, ataxia, sometimes hiccup, and bulbar symptoms. A few children have a head tilt to the side of the lesion. They occur more commonly in boys.

Modern treatment includes surgical removal of as much tumour as possible followed by cranial and spinal irradiation. Despite this there is a significant recurrence rate.

Cerebellar astrocytomas are slow growing relatively benign tumours which often can be completely excised. They present with cerebellar signs (page

80). *Ependymomas* may arise in the floor of the fourth ventricle and cause elevated ICP. The lower cranial nerves may be involved. Some arise supratentorially and many are calcified. Treatment is by surgery and radiotherapy but the prognosis is poor.

Adult Cerebral Tumours

Gliomas: these used to be described by cell type e.g. astrocytoma, but may be grouped together and divided into four grades based on their malignant activity (Kernohan), grade IV being the most malignant. Gliomas are invasive neoplasms often showing a variable content of malignancy within the tumour. Sometimes cystic, necrotic and even haemorrhagic areas are found in them. Commonly they are surrounded by an area of cerebral oedema. They are locally invasive and may spread across the corpus callosum. They carry a poor outlook although some are very slow growing. Some by their site may be totally resectable. The value of radiotherapy is debatable—in some patients life may be prolonged. Chemotherapy to date has proved disappointing.

Meningiomas: these may be asymptomatic but often present with focal signs and features of elevated ICP. Their common sites are parasagittal and falx (24%), these may invade the sagittal sinus, sphenoidal ridge (10%), convexity (18%), olfactory groove (10%), suprasellar (10%) and posterior fossa (10%). They are more common in women and very rarely undergo malignant change. Some calcify, producing changes on skull X-rays where they may also cause changes at the sites of their attachments to bone or enlarged middle meningeal feeding arteries. Such tumours should be surgically removed when causing symptoms. Some recur if incompletely removed and the value of radiotherapy in preventing recurrence is uncertain.

Pituitary tumours: these are usually locally invasive and cause headache, visual symptoms and disturbed endocrine functions (page 80). Occasionally they are very large and expand laterally into the cavernous sinus causing pain and ocular palsies, or even under the temporal lobe, frontal lobe or between the frontal lobes. The usual visual disturbance is bilateral loss of the temporal fields (two thirds) but in many patients this may be asymmetrical, or there may be loss of vision in one eye or the appearance of scotomatous field defects. Careful field charting is essential. With the use of radio-immuno-assays pituitary hormones can now be measured (HGH, TSH, LH, FSH, ACTH and prolactin) and the triple bolus test (page 21) will show if hypopituitarism is present.

In some patients there may be an *empty sella* (c. 10%) with an enlarged pituitary fossa containing no tumour. To avoid negative surgical exploration appropriate X-ray, visual and endocrine studies should always be made.

Pituitary apoplexy is the sudden haemorrhagic infarction of a pituitary tumour often accompanied by loss of consciousness, meningism and fever. Patients may show visual loss or an oculomotor palsy. The CSF is blood stained and xanthochromic.

Treatment of pituitary tumours involves a number of techniques. Very large tumours are best removed surgically through a frontal craniotomy. Smaller tumours can be more easily treated surgically by a trans-sphenoidal approach. This has a lower mortality and morbidity. Surgical treatment should be followed by radiotherapy which significantly reduces the recurrence rate, and by endocrine replacement therapy where indicated.

Other treatments include yttrium implants within the sella and external irradiation, the latter most effectively given by a proton beam (not widely available). These methods are not so effective and have problems, particularly radiation damage to the visual system.

Bromocriptine significantly lowers the secretion of growth hormone and prolactin and has been used to control tumours secreting these hormones.

Cerebral metastases: these are seen with greater frequency in general hospitals, particularly in the elderly. The common primary sources are from the bronchus, breast and kidney. Usually they are multiple (Plate 6) but occasionally single. Steroid treatment may produce temporary symptomatic relief.

Acoustic neuromas: these are benign tumours arising on the eighth nerve usually presenting with deafness, tinnitus, vertigo and unsteadiness. Hearing tests show a perceptive deafness with absence of loudness recruitment, and caloric tests a canal paresis. As the tumour enlarges medially, it compresses the brain stem and may produce hydrocephalus. The usual order of progression is eighth nerve involvement followed by trigeminal upset, commonly ophthalmic division sensory loss, then ipsilateral cerebellar signs followed by ocular symptoms and those of elevated ICP, then facial weakness and bulbar symptoms. About 5% of acoustic neuromas are bilateral.

Treatment is surgical often in a two stage operation aided by the operating microscope. Some surgeons combine a posterior fossa craniotomy with a translabyrinthine approach. A much lesser procedure is an intracapsular decompression but here there is a high recurrence rate. Often the facial nerve is damaged causing a persistent facial paralysis after surgery.

Vascular tumours: these include angiomas which commonly present with focal fits, an SAH or focal signs. Some patients have audible skull bruits and the malformation may be surgically accessible. Haemangioblastomas are commonly cystic arising in the cerebellum. They may be multiple and there is a familial incidence. If they are associated with retinal and spinal angiomas the term von Hippel-Lindau's disease may be used.

Investigations

These include plain X-rays of the skull (Plate 2a) and chest. Special views of certain sites may be indicated e.g. internal auditory canals or pituitary fossa (Plate 1), where tomography may also be helpful. Over 50% of cerebral tumours produce changes on the plain skull X-rays.

CT scanning will show most intracranial tumours, particularly if combined with contrast enhancement (Plates 3–6). CT scans will also show the presence of hydrocephalus and shifts or displacements of the ventricles and brain tissue. At certain sites, particularly in the para-sellar region, definition may not be sufficiently accurate on a CT scan to detect small masses e.g. a small supra-sellar pituitary extension, and here an AEG may be necessary. Vascular tumours such as angiomas (Plate 11b) may be well shown by angiography which will also give information about the blood supply of a tumour.

When CT scanning is not available isotope brain scans may show meningiomas (particularly supratentorial) and metastases but only about 50–60% of gliomas. They may not show lesions near the skull base or in the posterior fossa. If CT scanning is not available then angiography and an AEG or ventriculogram may still be necessary. AEGs may prove dangerous in the presence of raised ICP and here ventriculography prior to surgery may be a safer procedure. Such investigations should always be performed in conjunction with the neurosurgical team so more urgent surgical measures can be initiated if patients deteriorate.

Other investigations may be important; for example visual field charts and endocrine function tests in suspected pituitary tumours, and audiometry and caloric tests in suspected acoustic neuromas.

Elevated Intracranial Pressure (ICP)

This can be lowered by:

1. Reduction of oedema around the tumour—

(a) by hyperosmotic agents given intravenously. Mannitol in 20% solution, in adults 1–2 g/kg body weight, given over 15–20 minutes may be effective (page 57). It should be followed by other measures to continue the decompression as 'rebound' may occur. Urea (30% in 10% invert sugar in a dose of

1–1.5 g/kg body weight IV given over 20 minutes) has been used. Glycerol (1–2 g/kg body weight) can be given diluted orally or via a naso-gastric tube.

(b) by steroids. Dexamethasone 5 mg IV six hourly or 4 mg orally six hourly may be effective although slightly slower in onset.

2. Surgical decompression—

(a) Craniotomy with decompression. This is often combined with removal of as much tumour as is possible.

(b) Ventricular drainage of CSF through a ventriculo-atrial or ventriculo-peritoneal shunt. These combine a drainage tube, inserted through a burr hole in the skull into the lateral ventricle, connected via a one-way valve into the right atrium or peritoneal cavity. Unfortunately such shunts may become blocked, infected or even produce subdural haematomata.

Spinal Cord Compression

This may be a neurological emergency for after a time a critical state is reached where if compression continues, the blood supply to the cord may be cut off leaving irreversible damage, usually a paraplegia, loss of sensation below the level of damage and loss of sphincter control. Surgical decompression before this may allow full recovery. Table XIV indicates some of the more common causes of compression. The spinal cord ends usually at the level of the L1 disc in the adult so tumours below this level will compress the cauda equina.

Table XIV
Causes of Spinal Cord Compression

Tumours		
Benign	Neuroma	
	Meningioma	
Malignant	Metastases	
	Glioma	
	Ependymoma	
Infections	Extradural abscess (includes TB)	
Prolapsed intervertebral disc (PID)		
Trauma	Fracture-dislocation	
Haemorrhage	Anticoagulant treatment	
	Haemorrhagic diathesis	
Cysts	Arachnoid	
	Intramedullary—syrinx	
Skeletal deformity	Narrow canal	e.g. achondroplasia,
	Abnormal bone	Paget's, acromegaly

The symptoms and signs of cord compression depend on the site, the pathology and the speed of progression. Some medical conditions, as multiple sclerosis (MS), may mimic these features. Often at the level of compression there is involvement of nerve roots with pain and loss of function in the distribution of that root, and below that level upset motor, sensory and autonomic function in the spinal cord.

Motor disturbance commonly causes complaints of weakness, stiffness, or heaviness in the legs—sometimes mistaken for joint disease. These symptoms may be asymmetrical. In the cervical region there may also be weakness of the arms and hands, depending on the level. Usually there are signs of a spastic paraparesis with exaggerated leg reflexes and clonus, with extensor plantar responses. Often a reflex level is present with depressed or absent reflexes at the level of the lesion (involving the root or anterior horn cells) and increased reflexes below that level. On the trunk, the abdominal and cremasteric reflexes may help in determining a level. Weakness of the lower abdominal muscles may cause deviation of the umbilicus upwards on neck flexion, with lost lower abdominal reflexes.

Many patients are aware of *sensory upset* with numbness and tingling, sometimes feelings of cold, loss of temperature appreciation or other sensory functions. Patients may clearly indicate a level above which sensation is normal. Below there may be impairment of all sensory modalities. Sometimes compression seems to affect predominantly one side of the cord producing a Brown-Séquard syndrome. Here there is a spastic weakness with posterior column sensory loss on the side of the lesion, and spinothalamic (pain and temperature) sensory loss on the opposite side. This is due to the decussation of these fibres shortly after entering the cord. Compression high in the cervical region, above C3/4, may severely involve posterior columns producing marked sensory loss in the fingers, particularly joint position, with the appearance of pseudo-athetotic finger movements when the eyes are closed. With cervical lesions, neck flexion may cause pain or trigger electric-shock like sensations (Lhermitte's phenomenon) which radiate down the spine into the legs. This last most commonly occurs when plaques of demyelination appear in the posterior columns in the cervical region.

Autonomic symptoms produce sphincter disturbance with increasing constipation, or faecal soiling if diarrhoea is present. Urinary upset causes frequency and urgency of micturition, later retention with overflow incontinence; this may lead to catheterisation. By this stage cord compression is *critical* and needs urgent relief. In males there may be loss of potency. Retention may produce a palpable bladder and lesions at the level of the conus may produce a lax anal sphincter with loss of the anal reflex. Sensory function

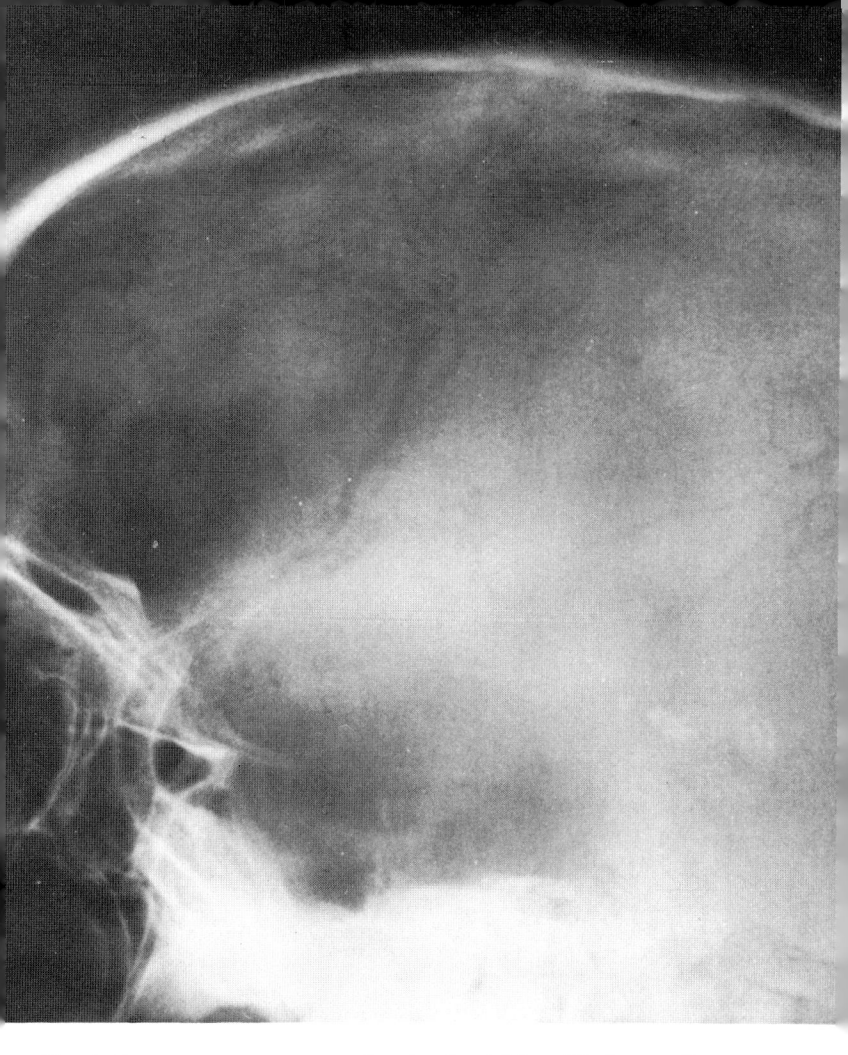

Plate 1: *Pituitary tumour causing an enlarged and eroded fossa. The dorsum sellae is barely visible.*

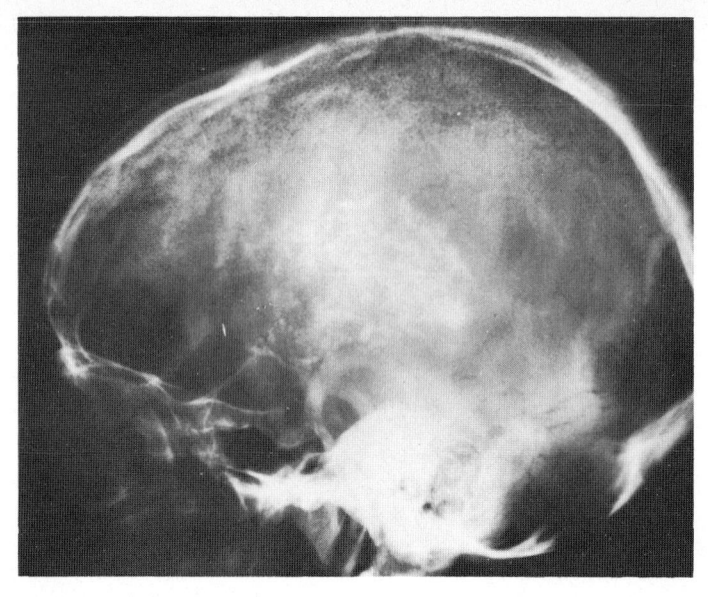

Plate 2a: *Lateral skull X-ray showing extensive calcification in a slow growing glioma.*

Plate 2b: *Lateral skull X-ray showing a ring of calcification in a large aneurysm in the frontal region.*

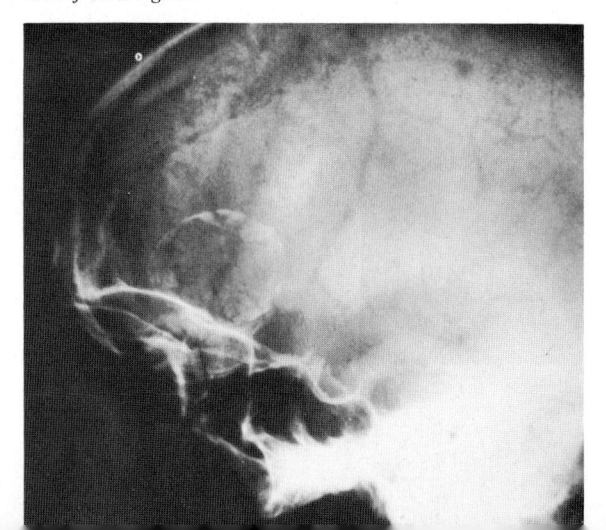

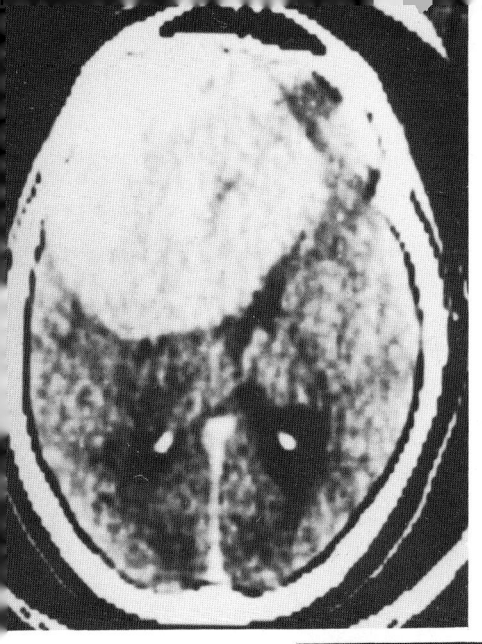

Plate 3a: *Enhanced CT brain scan showing a massive frontal meningioma.*

Plate 3b: *Enhanced CT brain scan showing a pituitary tumour with suprasellar extension spreading into the right frontal region.*

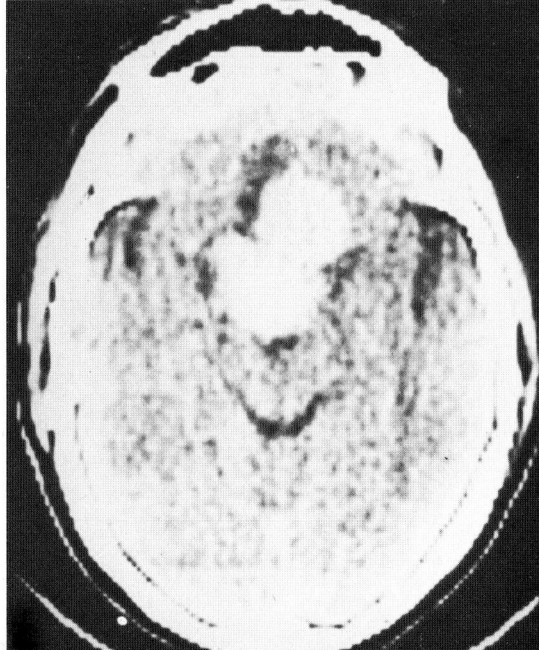

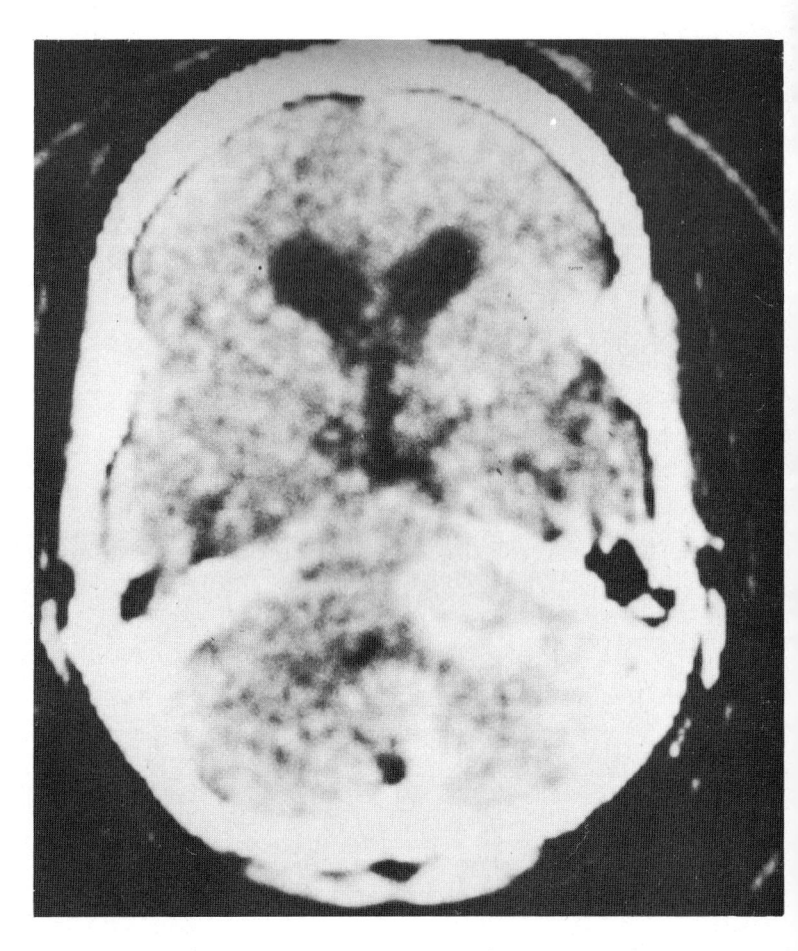

Plate 4: *Enhanced CT brain scan showing a right acoustic neuroma. The fourth ventricle is displaced to the left and the ventricles are slightly dilated.*

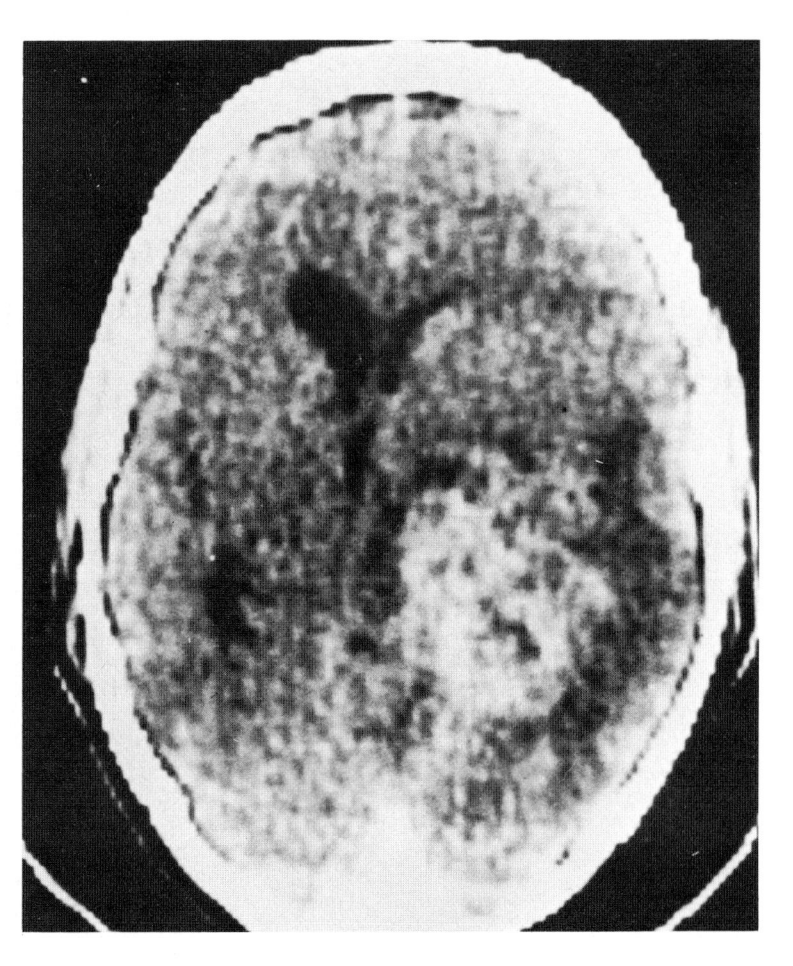

Plate 5: *Enhanced CT brain scan showing an extensive glioma in the right parieto-temporal region. There is surrounding oedema and compression of the right lateral ventricle.*

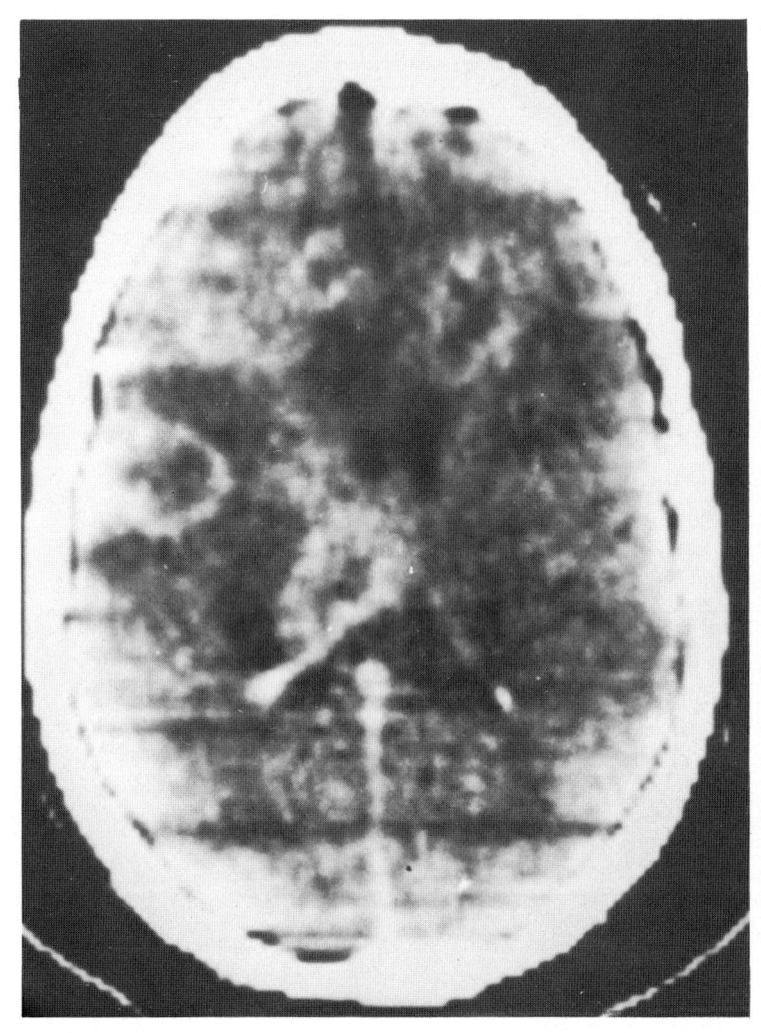

Plate 6: *Enhanced CT brain scan showing multiple metastases. There is some movement artefact.*

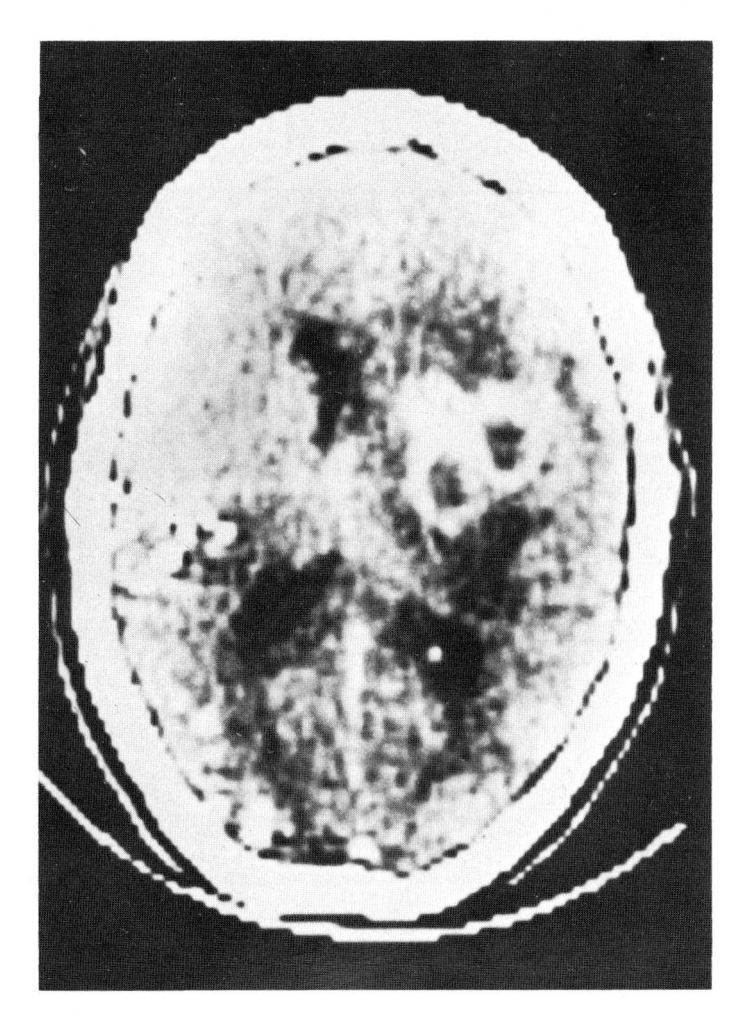

Plate 7: *Enhanced CT brain scan showing a biloculated abscess in the right thalamic region. There is surrounding oedema and shift of mid-line structures.*

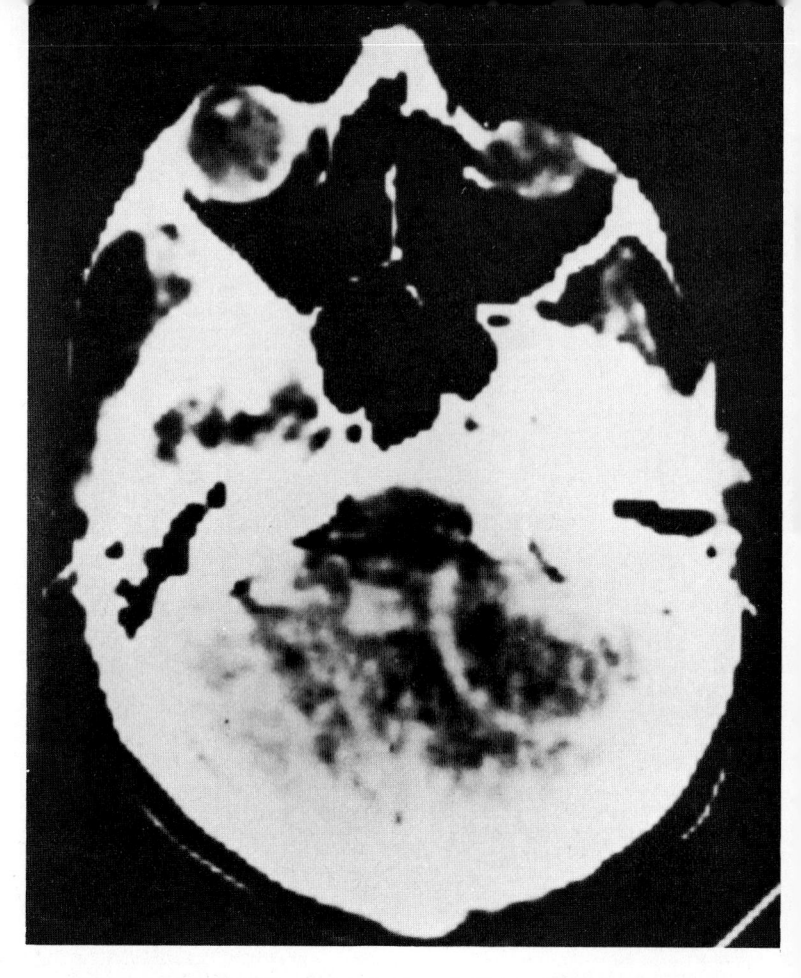

Plate 8: *Enhanced CT brain scan showing a half ring of high density outlining a lesion in the right cerebello-pontine angle. This was a right cerebellar abscess.*

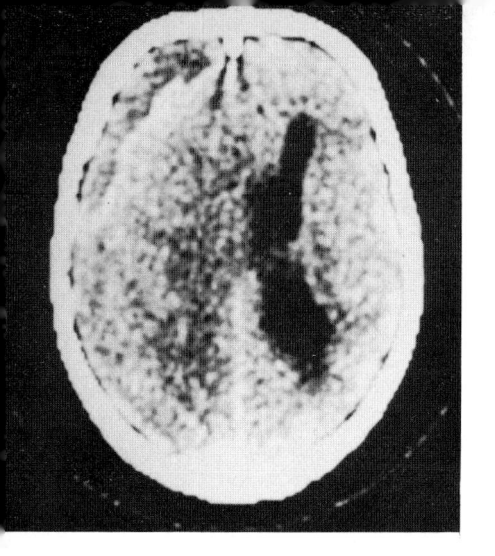

Plate 9a: *CT brain scan showing a subdural haematoma causing marked shift so the left lateral ventricle is poorly seen and the right dilated.*

Plate 9b: *CT brain scan showing a wedge-shaped area of low density in the left parieto-temporal region and two smaller areas in the right hemisphere. These were infarcts.*

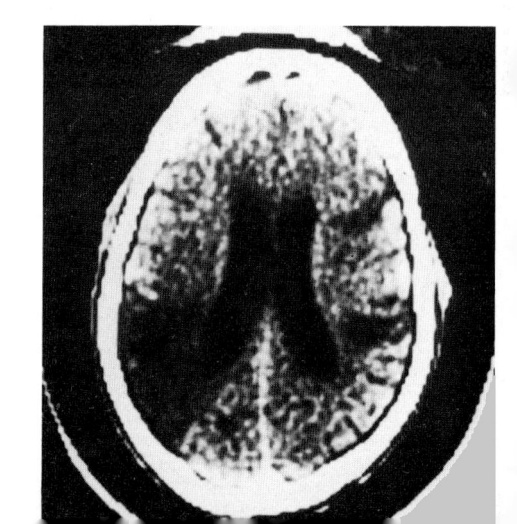

Plate 10a: *CT brain scan in an unconscious patient showing a high density lesion in the left hemisphere causing considerable shift. This was an intracerebral haematoma.*

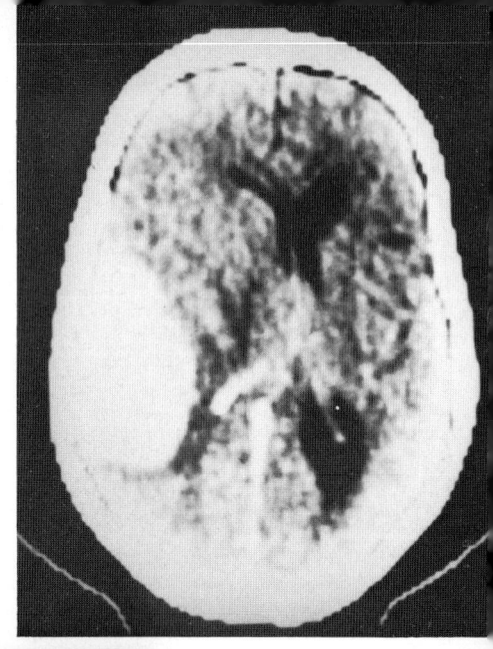

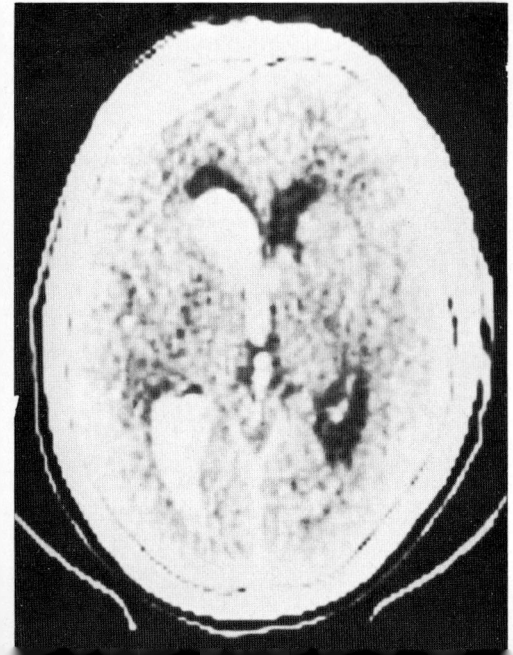

Plate 10b: *CT brain scan showing blood (high density) in the left lateral and third ventricles. This was caused by an SAH from a ruptured aneurysm.*

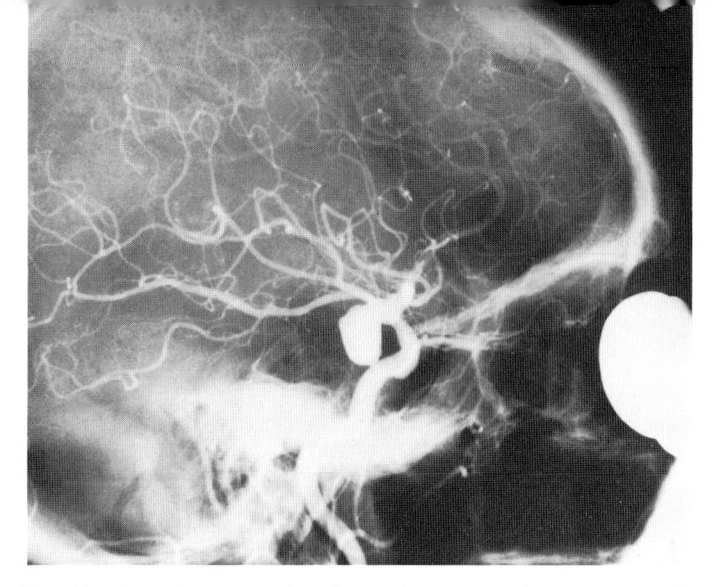

Plate 11a: *Carotid angiogram (lateral view) showing a very large aneurysm at the termination of the internal carotid artery.*

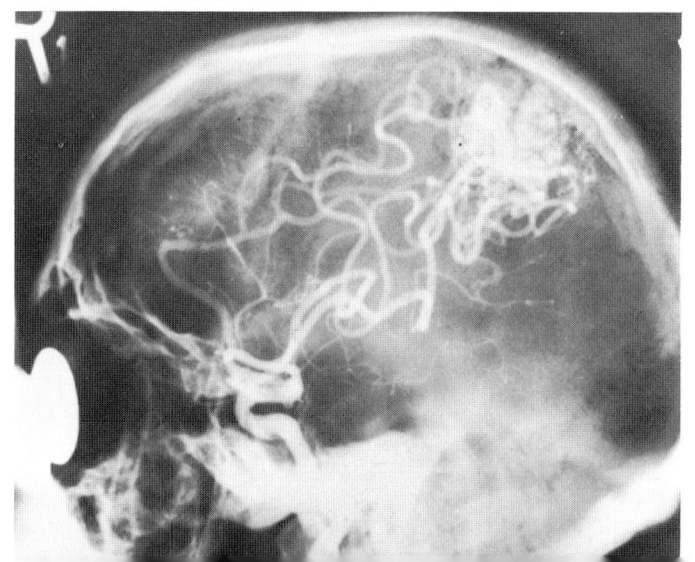

Plate 11b: *Carotid angiogram (lateral view) showing an angioma.*

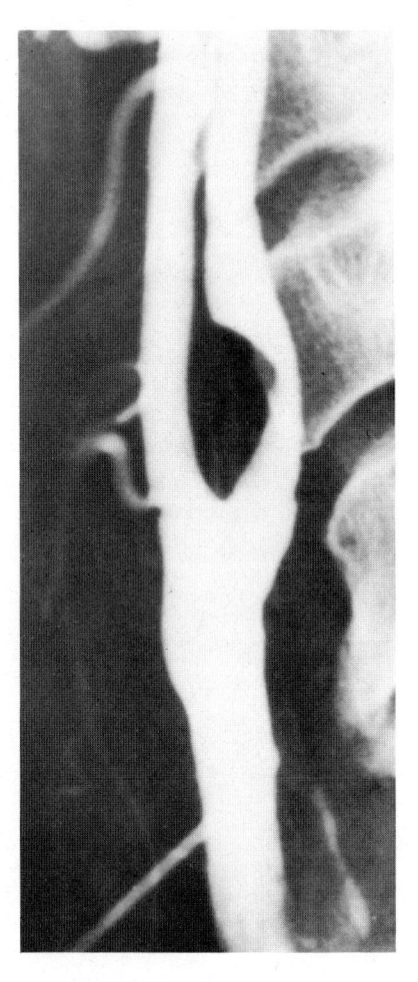

Plate 12: *Common carotid angiogram (the needle is seen) showing a stenotic lesion at the origin of the internal carotid artery.*

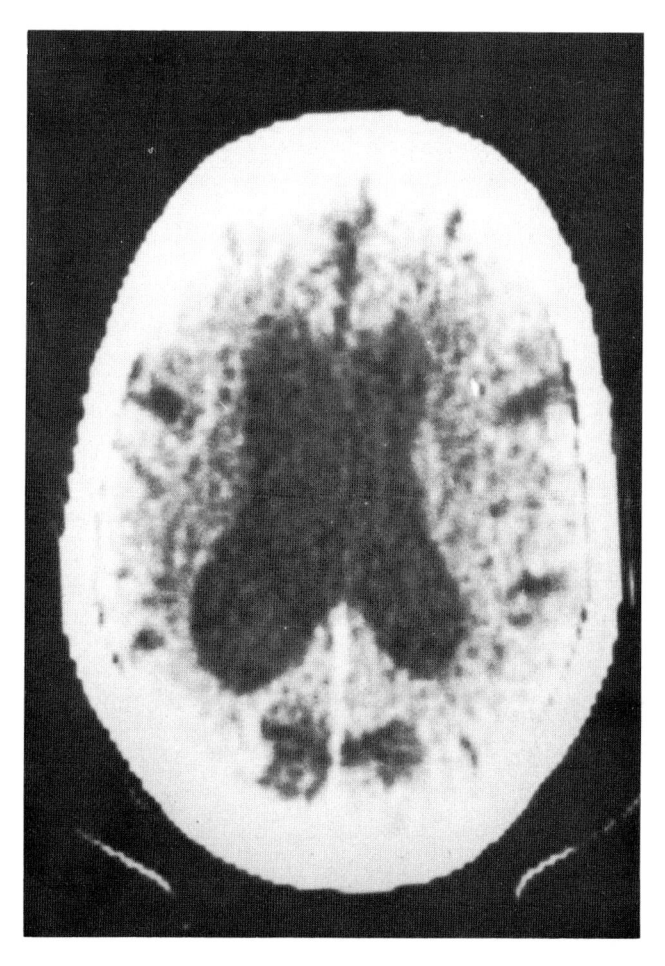

Plate 13: *CT brain scan showing marked ventricular dilation and patchy areas of low density prominent in the occipital lobes. This patient had a multi-infarct dementia.*

Plate 14a: *Metrizamide myelogram (lateral view) showing complete block in the mid-thoracic region with a rounded contour. This was a meningioma.*

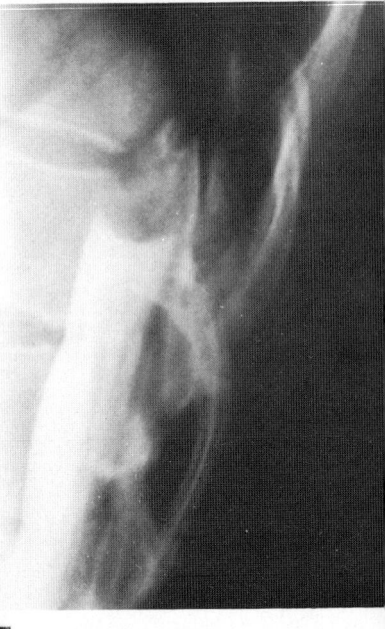

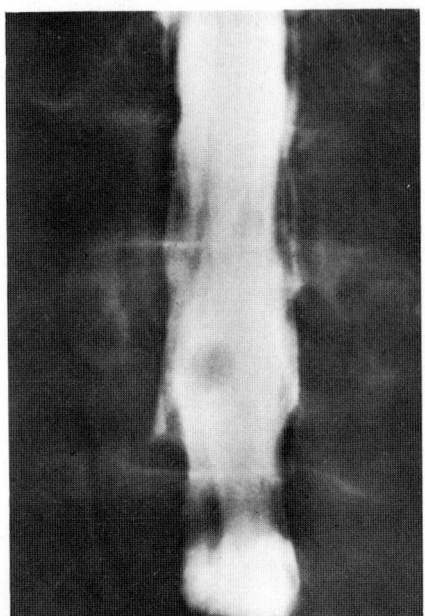

Plate 14b: *Metrizamide radiculogram showing a neuroma on a lumbar root.*

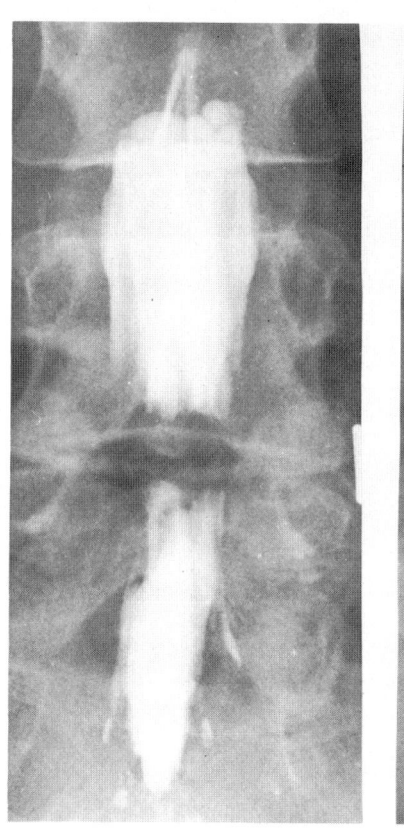

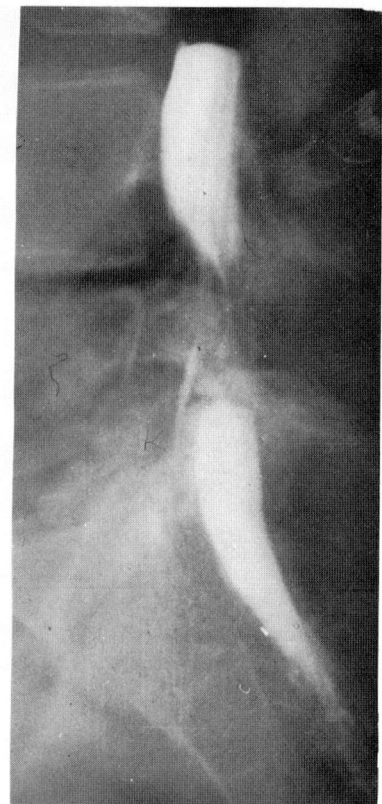

Plate 15: *Myelogram (PA and lateral views) showing a large central disc prolapse at L 4/5.*

Plate 16a: *Myelogram (PA view) showing an expanded spinal cord in the cervical region caused by an intramedullary tumour.*

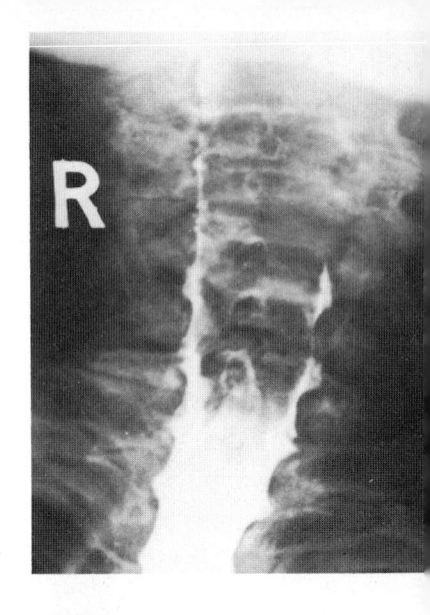

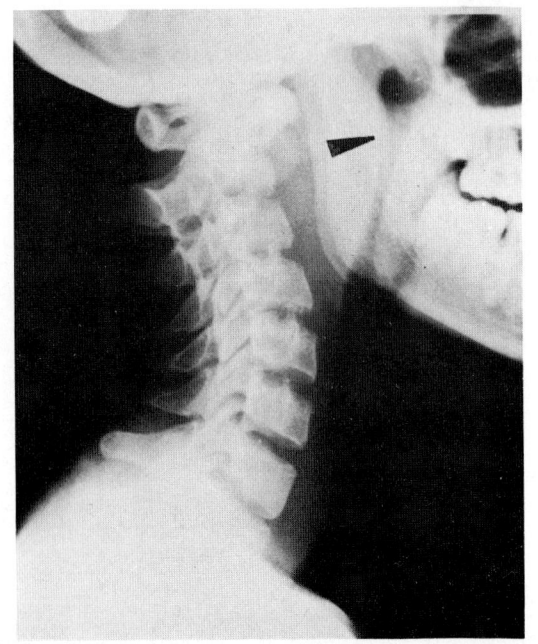

Plate 16b: *Lateral view of t cervical spine showing atlant axial subluxation. A promine soft tissue swelling (arrowed) seen at the back of the throat. T was a retro-pharyngeal tuberc lous abscess.*

SPINAL CORD COMPRESSION

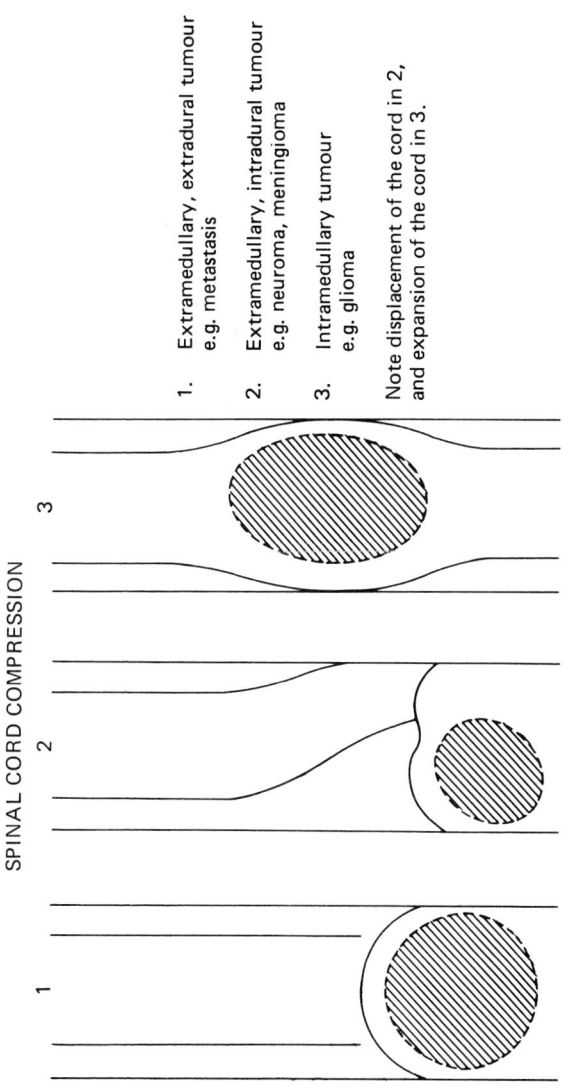

1. Extramedullary, extradural tumour e.g. metastasis
2. Extramedullary, intradural tumour e.g. neuroma, meningioma
3. Intramedullary tumour e.g. glioma

Note displacement of the cord in 2, and expansion of the cord in 3.

Figure 4: *Myelographic Appearances of Spinal Cord Compression*

in the lower sacral segments should always be checked; intramedullary lesions are said sometimes to produce sparing of sacral sensation in an area of distal sensory loss.

Abscesses and tumours causing cord compression often produce local *spinal pain* aggravated by movement and weight bearing. The pain may spread in a girdle distribution along the course of an affected root. Stiffness or restricted spinal movements may be apparent, and these may cause a scoliosis. Back pain worse while resting in bed is more likely to be caused by a tumour than a prolapsed intervertebral disc (PID). A narrow spinal canal is more likely to be associated with cord compression and occasionally symptoms may be intermittent, provoked by exercise and eased by rest (e.g. cauda equina claudicans). A parasagittal lesion may cause a spastic paraparesis.

Investigations

These include an FBC, ESR, urea, electrolytes, blood glucose, and WR +. In patients with a paraparesis, blood should also be sent for a B_{12} estimation. If metastatic deposits could be responsible a chest X-ray, serum proteins and 'strip', calcium and acid and alkaline phosphatases should be included.

Good quality plain X-rays of the spine may give the answer but they must be taken at the appropriate level. Tomograms at that level may give further detail. If there is a clear sensory level, then it is likely that the cord lesion responsible lies three to four segments higher. Pedicle erosion, changes in bone density, vertebral body collapse, malalignments or paraspinal soft tissue shadows may be present (Plate 16b).

A myelogram with CSF examination is the important investigation. This will show a compressive lesion, and often indicate its nature (Fig. 4, Plate 14a). At the time of the lumbar puncture to introduce contrast medium, a manometric block may be demonstrated by no pressure change on coughing or compression of the jugular veins. It is worth asking the radiologist to leave a marker on the skin at the level of any block so that the surgeon knows the correct level of the compressive lesion. It is wise to try to introduce the contrast medium below the suspected level of compression. Occasionally, it may be necessary to inject it from above by cisternal puncture (a procedure only for experts).

Surgical decompression should always be undertaken providing patients can withstand operation and the cord damage is still reversible. Even extradural metastases should be decompressed as this affords a better quality of survival without leg paralysis or sphincter loss. During recovery active physiotherapy may be a major help. Long lesions may necessitate a widespread decompression and in certain types of tumour, radiotherapy and chemotherapy may be necessary.

13. SPINAL DEGENERATIVE DISEASE

Prolapsed Intervertebral Disc

The diameter of the spinal canal varies. Patients with congenitally narrowed canals are more likely to develop cord or root compression if they prolapse an intervertebral disc (PID). Furthermore with increasing age, the bony surfaces roughen and osteophytic spurs appear which may protrude into the exit foramina. The lining ligaments may hypertrophy narrowing the spinal canal further. In certain conditions the canal may also narrow, e.g. Paget's disease, acromegaly, achondroplasia. Rare degenerative diseases may cause instability of the spinal joints which may lead to cord compression, e.g. atlanto-axial subluxation in patients with rheumatoid arthritis.

The commonest sites of spinal cord and root compression from degenerative disease lie in the cervical and lumbar regions. The maximum incidence of PID in the *lumbar region* is at L5/S1 (S1 root), and the next most frequent level is at L4/5 (L5 root). Usually the protrusion arises laterally, compressing a single root causing sciatica with pain in the distribution of the myotome and tingling and numbness in the distribution of the dermatome. The pain is aggravated by measures that elevate intrathecal pressure, e.g. cough. As compression continues, weakness and sensory loss may develop, often with a depressed or absent reflex. The distribution of the signs depends on the level involved (Fig. 2). Many patients give a past history of recurrent backache, lumbago, often accompanied by attacks of sciatica. An acute exacerbation may be provoked by lifting, straining or sudden movement.

Examining patients with acute sciatica may be complicated by pain which produces muscle spasm making assessment of power difficult. Furthermore some roots which may be involved, e.g. L5, may have no reflex signs, and because of the overlap of dermatomes, sensory loss may be minimal. However the distribution of sensory symptoms often indicates which root is compressed.

In most instances, *root tension signs* will be present with restricted straight leg raising, the pain being aggravated by ankle dorsiflexion with the knee extended. L3 root lesions, which are uncommon, may produce a positive femoral stretch test—limitation of extension of the hip with patients lying prone.

Discs may also herniate centrally compressing a number of nerve roots usually producing bilateral symptoms and signs, sacral numbness and sphincter upset (through involvement of the sacral roots). Central disc protrusions with sphincter upset should be treated as an emergency to avoid permanent damage to the nerves. Such patients should be admitted urgently to a neurosurgical unit with a view to immediate myelography and decompression.

Cervical roots may also be irritated or compressed by a lateral disc protrusion or bony osteophytic spurs. Most commonly C6, C7 and C5 are involved. Here again severe pain is produced in the distribution of the affected root with later weakness, sensory loss and reflex changes. Pain is common in the neck radiating to the shoulder and may be aggravated by neck movements. It should be emphasised that lateral flexion of the neck tests movements of the cervical intervertebral joints; lateral rotation and flexion and extension take place at the atlanto-axial and cranio-cervical junctions.

A central cervical disc protrusion will compress the cord producing a myelopathy often with symptoms and signs of involvement of the motor and sensory tracts to the legs and some sphincter upset (page 86). Usually at the level of compression in the neck, one root is involved with local signs and a depressed or absent arm reflex.

Investigations

An acute radiculopathy requires investigation: most commonly this is produced by a PID. Roots may also be compressed by tumours, become acutely inflamed e.g. neuralgic amyotrophy (page 92), or infected e.g. zoster (page 51), or disturbed by metabolic upset e.g. diabetic amyotrophy (page 92).

Blood should be taken for an FBC, ESR, blood glucose, WR+, and if cord signs are present for a serum B_{12} level.

Good quality plain X-rays of the affected part of the spine will support a diagnosis of degenerative spinal disease showing narrowed disc spaces, irregular bony edges and a narrowed canal. However one of the difficulties is that in many older patients, degenerative changes may be present on X-ray even when patients are symptom-free. Other pathology may be indicated by X-ray changes, e.g. pedicle erosion or a paraspinal soft tissue swelling (Plate 16b). A disc prolapse may produce no X-ray change so myelography is necessary. This is particularly important if other diagnoses need exclusion and there are signs of cord involvement. Many radiologists now prefer metrizamide which is water-soluble and gives excellent pictures in the lumbar region. Most significant disc prolapses are well shown (Plate 15) but if there is a wide space between the backs of the vertical bodies (usually at L5/S1) and the theca, a disc protrusion may still be present which may not show clearly.

CSF taken at the time of myelography may be normal in patients with a PID; often the protein is mildly elevated. This elevation may be higher if cord compression has occurred.

Treatment

Treatment of a disc protrusion is in most instances initially by *medical means*. Lumbar disc lesions often respond to three to four weeks strict bed-rest on a firm mattress accompanied by regular doses of analgesics and muscle relaxants (e.g. diazepam). This may be followed by mobilisation aided by physiotherapy, e.g. lumbar isometric extension exercises, when the severe pain has settled. In some patients the back may need more prolonged support in a corset or plaster jacket.

Cervical disc lesions may also respond to similar measures. Although many doctors recommend support in a firm collar, if pain is severe and acute, many patients respond better to strict bed-rest with sufficient analgesia. Again as the pain eases, physiotherapy will prove beneficial with heat and exercises. At this stage support in a firm collar for four to six weeks may help.

Traction, either for lumbar discs applied to the legs, or for cervical root lesions applied to the head, has its advocates. Some patients benefit.

In patients where progressive neurological deficit appears, where there is diagnostic doubt as to the cause, where conservative measures have failed to give relief, or where there are frequent recurring episodes, myelography should be performed with a view to surgical decompression of any significant sized lesion. If a single cervical root is compressed, a foraminotomy may be performed. In the neck where root and cord compression occurs at a single level, an anterior approach to the disc prolapse with its excision followed by bone grafting (Cloward's procedure) may be used. If there is widespread compression, often at several levels, then a posterior decompressive laminectomy may be the choice. In the lumbar region, a laminectomy with excision of the protruded disc may be necessary. Surgical exploration of patients with normal myelograms seldom relieves pain.

Manipulation is widely practised by osteopaths often with good relief of back pain. Manipulation by doctors may be very effective in the relief of pain but such treatment may aggravate the pain and signs if there is actual root compression from a large disc fragment or if the diagnosis is incorrect. If a central protrusion is suspected, manipulation is contra-indicated.

Other Painful Root Lesions

These include:

1. **Herpes zoster** (page 51).

2. **Neuralgic amyotrophy**: this causes severe pain in the shoulder radiating into the arm. The pain usually subsides within two to three weeks leaving signs of weakness which are often patchy, i.e. not only affecting muscles supplied by a single root. There is commonly wasting, reflex loss at affected levels and often some sensory impairment. In over 50% signs are confined to the shoulder girdles but in nearly one third there may be bilateral involvement. Rarely there may be recurrent attacks.

The CSF is often normal. EMG studies may show evidence of denervation in affected muscles. Most patients recover fully but if denervation has occurred recovery may be slow (two years). It is thought to be due to an acute inflammation of part of the brachial plexus perhaps secondary to a viral infection. In about one third there is a history of antecedent respiratory infection and in some patients it has followed immunisation.

3. **Diabetic amyotrophy**: more correctly this is a femoral neuropathy causing acute severe pain in the thigh, often worse at night. It is associated with weakness, wasting of the thigh and a depressed or absent knee reflex. Often there is weakness of hip flexion. There may be an area of sensory loss on the thigh. In many patients there are also more distal neuropathic signs with lost ankle jerks and impaired vibratory sense in the feet. It may be the presenting symptom of undiagnosed diabetes.

In many patients the CSF protein is elevated. EMG studies will confirm denervation in thigh muscles often with a prolonged latency in the femoral nerve. In most patients recovery occurs with good control of the diabetes. The cause has been shown as due to an infarction of the femoral nerve.

4. **Carcinomatous root compression**

Note also that many *entrapment syndromes* cause referred pain in the limbs, e.g. carpal tunnel syndrome.

Syringomyelia

This is an uncommon condition where cavitation occurs within the spinal cord, usually in the cervical region. Rarely it extends caudally and sometimes up into the medulla (syringobulbia). It may occur secondary to trauma or a spinal tumour but more often is linked with a developmental abnormality at the cranio-cervical junction. Here the cerebellar tonsils herniate through the foramen magnum compressing the upper cord and produce a block. Probably secondary to this, pressure waves force the CSF into the central canal of the cord which gradually expands producing symptoms and signs of a central cord lesion.

Usually there are complaints of gradually increasing weakness and wasting of the small hand muscles. The reflexes in the arms are depressed or lost. Sensory symptoms may be the presenting feature with the development of painless injuries in the hands from spinothalamic sensory loss. The sensory loss is dissociated for the posterior columns are spared. Trophic skin changes may occur in affected areas and c. 20% of patients develop neuropathic joints. Later the long tracts to the legs may be involved with the development of spastic weakness, sphincter upset and sensory signs.

X-rays of the cervical spine may show a widened canal and myelography will show an expanded cord often with tonsillar herniation (supine screening). The upper cervical roots appear to travel horizontally. CT scanning may show a degree of hydrocephalus. The CSF protein may be elevated particularly if there is a block.

In younger patients with progressive deterioration, surgical decompression at the foramen magnum may arrest progress. Such procedures are sometimes combined with attempts to occlude the upper end of the central canal. Hydrocephalus may be treated by shunting. In older patients or those with static disease, conservative management is often possible.

14. DEMYELINATING DISEASES

Multiple Sclerosis

Demyelination causes patchy loss of the myelin sheath in nerve fibres in the CNS. The commonest cause is multiple sclerosis (MS) but rarely it may also occur after certain infections e.g. measles, chicken pox, or following smallpox vaccination. In MS, scattered perivenous foci of inflammation appear in the white matter. Almost any part of the CNS may be involved but most commonly lesions appear in the spinal cord (in the posterior, lateral and intermedio-lateral columns), in the mid-brain, pons and cerebellar peduncles, in the optic nerves and in the periventricular white matter in the hemispheres.

The cause of MS is unknown although many theories have been suggested. Because of this there is no specific diagnostic test that is completely reliable, and there is no effective cure. MS is a clinical diagnosis and may mimic other conditions e.g. spinal cord compression. The diagnosis rests on the exclusion of other possibilities coupled with evidence of dissemination of lesions anatomically and occurring at different times.

MS has a high incidence in cold temperate climates ($>30°$ latitude). It affects women more than men with a maximum age incidence in the third decade. The first attack in many patients may be mild and can be missed unless specific inquiry is made.

Clinically the condition usually follows a pattern of acute relapses and remissions. In many early attacks full recovery may occcur but with increasing time many patients are left with residual deficits which may increase with successive relapses, usually culminating in a severely disabled patient (often paraplegic with lost sphincter control).

Presentation

Patients may present with a single symptom or many symptoms. *Weakness* in one or both legs is common often with the appearance of a spastic foot drop. Patients may complain of trouble in one leg and on examination have signs in both legs—a spastic paraparesis with posterior column sensory disturbance. Sometimes cord plaques may produce a clear sensory level on the trunk. *Sensory disturbances* in the trunk and limbs may be described as 'tight bands' or other abnormal feelings—'cold water trickling, tingling, numbness, or burning'. In some patients cord lesions may present as a slowly progressive spastic weakness of the legs. This is more common in middle aged patients, particularly men.

A plaque in the posterior columns in the cervical region may produce marked sensory loss in the hand—lost position sense and discriminative function, which may render the hand 'useless'. Symptoms are often bilateral and may be accompanied by pyramidal signs. Lhermitte's phenomenon (neck flexion producing tingling or 'electric shocks' radiating down the spine to the legs or into the arms) may occur with plaques in the posterior columns in the neck. Although this is common in MS, it may also occur with other pathology.

Disturbances of the intermedio-lateral columns may cause *sphincter upset* with increasing constipation, and usually urgency and frequency of micturition. Later hesitancy, retention and incontinence may occur. In males impotence may occur.

Lesions within the brain stem may produce *visual disturbances*, sometimes diplopia. Involvement of the abducens and oculomotor nerves may appear but more often there is a bilateral internuclear ophthalmoplegia (page 8) with upset conjugate gaze from side to side. Many patients complain of facial sensory upset and may show facial weakness (LMN type), often erroneously labelled a Bell's palsy. The appearance of trigeminal neuralgia in a young patient may be the presentation of MS. The commonest brain stem disorder is that of cerebellar upset with ataxia of stance and gait, often with limb inco-ordination, dysarthria and nystagmus. Acute vertigo with vomiting may occur with brain stem plaques. In many patients there are associated cerebellar signs and often long tract signs. Deafness is relatively uncommon.

Optic nerve involvement leads to the development of optic neuritis. This may occur in isolation but in careful follow up studies of patients who present with optic neuritis, over 50% develop MS at a later date.

Acute involvement of one optic nerve causes depression of visual acuity. This may be mild or severe and is accompanied by visual field loss—usually a central scotoma. Pain may be felt in the affected eye, aggravated by eye movement. There is an afferent pupillary defect (page 6) and impaired colour vision. In the acute stage, the optic disc may appear normal unless the lesion is far forward on the papilla, a papillitis, when the nerve head may appear swollen. Following an acute episode of optic neuritis, 90% of patients have good recovery of vision (at least to 6/9), but in many there may be slight residual depression of acuity, impaired colour vision, an afferent pupillary defect, and disc pallor (optic atrophy).

Features of *cerebral hemisphere involvement* are most commonly related to mental changes. Patients may appear euphoric or depressed. Many with long-standing disease appear demented. The appearance of a hemianopia or hemiplegia is rare. MS patients have an increased incidence of fits. They may also show paroxysmal disorders as dysarthria or sensory symptoms.

Diagnosis

Diagnosis is largely clinical, excluding other causes. Certain tests may support the diagnosis although none are pathognomonic.

Routine *CSF examination* may show an increased cell count, usually $5-30$ lymphocytes/mm^3 in c. 25%. A mild protein rise is found in c. 30%—$0.4-1.0$ g/l. This is due to a rise in the gamma globulin fraction and if this is measured and expressed as a percentage of the total CSF protein then c. $80-85$% of MS patients have an IgG value of >20%. However certain other conditions may also cause a high IgG value e.g. neurosyphilis. By the use of polyacrilamide gel electrophoresis it has been possible to show an oligoclonal band of IgG in the CSF of c.90% of MS patients (Thompson *et al.*, 1979).

Electrophysiological studies can be used to show where demyelination has damaged nervous pathways (either current or past) for there is delay in impulse conduction. VERs (page 25) are commonly measured and significant delay suggests visual pathway involvement. Normal values vary amongst different laboratories but a wide difference in latency between the two eyes or a major delay indicates damage. Again such delay can be caused by conditions other than MS. However in certain patients, where for example there are signs of a spastic paraparesis and no past history of note, the presence of abnormal VERs indicates anatomical dissemination and may prevent further invasive neuroradiological investigations.

In some centres, auditory evoked responses and spinal and cortical somatosensory evoked responses may give an indication of damage in these pathways. Other electrophysiological studies include measurements of saccadic velocities of eye movements with electronystagmography to show slowing in patients with MS.

There has also been interest in determining HLA antigen patterns in patients with MS (in Great Britain HLA DRw2 are common). Claims have been made of specific diagnostic serological tests using the red cells of MS patients but such work has not been well substantiated and no simple laboratory test exists.

In many patients the diagnosis becomes apparent with follow up.

Treatment

There is no known cure for MS but there is good evidence that in an acute relapse a course of steroids may hasten recovery, although they will not alter the degree of that recovery. ACTH may be given by daily injection—80, 40 and 20 units, each dose given for seven days. Dexamethasone and prednisolone have also been used. Long term steroid treatment produces no benefit.

In a severe acute relapse rest is important. Intercurrent infections should be treated as sometimes they are responsible for the relapse, e.g. an occult urinary infection. Physiotherapy may be very helpful in restoring mobility.

In time progressive disability often appears with marked leg weakness so patients may be confined to wheel-chairs. At this stage help may be necessary in the provision of aids and home adaptations. Symptomatic treatment for various problems may be helpful, e.g. propantheline may reduce urgency and frequency of micturition, carbamazepine may be useful in controlling paroxysmal disturbances.

Spasticity, usually producing flexion in the legs with later contractures, may prove painful and troublesome. It may respond to diazepam, dantrolene sodium, or baclofen. Treatment is started in low dosage and slowly built up.

In severely disabled paraplegic or tetraplegic patients special care of the skin is necessary. Good nutrition and correction of anaemia are important. The best management of incontinent patients remains undecided: long term catheterisation creates problems but drainage appliances in the femal are not successful.

Many claims for treatment of MS have been made; these have not withstood clinical trial. They include long term steroid treatment, a gluten-free diet, and giving polyunsaturated fatty acids. In the last group some possible reduction in the duration and severity of relapses occurred if high doses were used, but overall improvement was not found.

Neuromyelitis Optica (Devic's syndrome)

This describes acute demyelination affecting both optic nerves and the spinal cord. In the latter there is a transverse myelitis; acute inflammation 'transecting' the spinal cord. The optic nerve and cord involvement may follow each other or occur together. In a proportion of patients, symptoms and signs of demyelination at other sites in the CNS appear subsequently.

Acute visual loss

A significant number of patients may have an episode of optic neuritis which occurs in isolation. The features may be identical to those described. Rarely local infections or even compressive lesions may cause acute visual loss. This may affect one or both eyes. Causes include acute sinus infections, a mucocoele of the sphenoid sinus, a cavernous sinus thrombosis, an aneurysm on the top of the internal carotid artery or from a pituitary tumour. Occasionally other tumours involving the chiasm or optic nerves may be responsible. In elderly patients vascular lesions of the optic nerve may occur: giant cell arteritis always should be excluded.

In such patients the visual acuity and fields should be serially charted. An FBC, ESR, WR+ and X-rays of the skull, orbits, optic foramina and chest should be made. A CT brain scan with views of the orbits and optic nerves, and sometimes angiography or even an AEG may be necessary. VERs and electroretinograms, and tests of pituitary function may be indicated. CSF examination is often necessary. A temporal artery biopsy or fluorescein retinal angiogram may need to be performed. Often joint consultation with an ophthalmologist may be helpful.

15. DEGENERATIVE DISORDERS

Dementia

With increasing age, many patients show some decline of their higher intellectual functions. In some this becomes apparent too early—a presenile dementia. Such patients may present with rather non-specific complaints of malaise, headache, dizziness, or a 'muzzy head'. More commonly relatives, work-mates or even teachers may comment on deterioration in their mental performance. Complaints of difficulty with memory, the ability to cope at home or in business, or in decision making, may be accompanied by changes in behaviour. Later physical deterioration may become apparent with neglect of personal hygiene and incontinence. In some patients depression may be the presenting symptom.

Many such patients have degenerative brain disease with progressive neuronal loss. The cause for this is often unknown and currently no treatment is effective. However in about 15% of patients presenting with dementia there is a treatable cause. Common causes are shown in Table XV.

In patients with dementia it is essential to interview relatives and to obtain a psychometric assessment (page 5).

Investigations: these include an FBC, ESR, thyroxine, WR + , serum B_{12}, and X-rays of the skull and chest. Where appropriate a serum calcium, liver function tests, urea and electrolytes may be added. A CT scan will show the presence of structural changes as atrophy, a tumour or hydrocephalus. As it is impossible to scan all elderly patients some selection is necessary but all young patients should be included. An EEG may be very helpful: it may show a diffuse or focal upset and in a few rare instances, e.g. Jakob-Creutzfeldt's disease, the appearance may be diagnostic. In selected patients the CSF should be examined. If a communicating hydrocephalus is suspected, a RIHSA scan may also be necessary in addition to a CT scan. An AEG may show atrophy or suggest a communicating hydrocephalus if CT scanning is not available.

Alzheimer's disease is the commonest cause of presenile dementia. It causes diffuse neuronal degeneration affecting the cerebral cortex, the brunt falling on the frontal lobes. The brain becomes atrophic and histologically resembles a senile brain. Patients present between the ages of 40–60 with

Table XV
Causes of Dementia

1. Degenerative neuronal loss
    i. Alzheimer's disease
    ii. Huntington's chorea
    iii. Steele-Richardson-Olszewski's syndrome
    iv. Tuberose sclerosis
2. Infective
    i. Post meningo-encephalitis
    ii. 'Slow' viral infection, Jakob-Creutzfeldt
    iii. Neurosyphilis
3. Trauma
    Brain damage, chronic subdural haematoma
4. Inflammatory
    Multiple sclerosis
5. Tumours
    i. Direct invasion frontal and temporal lobes, corpus callosum
    ii. With obstructive hydrocephalus
    iii. Multiple metastases
    iv. Carcinomatous meningitis
6. Metabolic
    i. B_{12} deficit
    ii. B_1 deficit (Wernicke's encephalopathy)
    iii. Myxoedema
    iv. Post prolonged hypoglycaemia
    v. Hypercalcaemia
    vi. Dialysis
7. Poisoning
    Barbiturates, alcohol
8. Communicating Hydrocephalus
9. Vascular
    i. Multi-infarct dementia
    ii. Angioma with 'steal'
    iii. Post 'stroke'
    iv. Post subarachnoid haemorrhage
10. Anoxic
    After cardiac arrest, CO poisoning, respiratory failure

---

initially failing memory, impaired performance and spatial disorientation. Later there are difficulties with reading, writing and speaking, and there may be an apraxia. Physical deterioration follows: patients becoming slow, apathetic, bed-ridden and incontinent. They may show a mixture of pyramidal and extrapyramidal signs with exaggerated reflexes and extensor plantar responses. Primitive reflexes may be prominent with brisk pout, suck, 'rooting' and facial reflexes often combined with grasp and palmo-mental reflexes. Fits may occur. Most patients die two to five years after the diagnosis.

Huntington's chorea is an autosomal dominant inherited disorder where a progressive dementia is accompanied by choreiform involuntary movements. The frontal lobes and putamen show extensive nerve cell loss accompanied by gliosis. The onset is usually between the ages of 25–40, and may present with mental symptoms, e.g. emotional upsets, dementia, paranoia, or with involuntary movements, clumsiness and poor balance. Patients survive for a long time with a mean duration of c. 15 years, most ending as inmates of mental hospitals. Occasionally they present in childhood with rigidity, tremor, ataxia and mental retardation. Recognition is important for genetic counselling.

The choreic movements may be improved by phenothiazines (e.g. thiopropazate), butyrophenones (e.g. haloperidol), or tetrabenazine.

Jakob-Creutzfeldt's disease has aroused recent interest for it can be transmitted to animals confirming that it is due to a viral infection with a very long latency ('slow virus'). It produces a rapidly progressive dementia, many patients dying between 9–24 months from the onset. Histologically the brain shows neuronal loss with marked astrocytic proliferation and frequently a curious spongy appearance—status spongiosus (spongiform encephalopathy). The damage affects different sites to a variable degree accounting for the widely variable clinical presentations.

Patients are usually aged 40–60 and early symptoms include non-specific malaise, fatiguability, memory impairment, slowing-up and behaviour changes. The gait becomes unsteady, and pyramidal, extrapyramidal and cerebellar signs appear. Tremor, choreic movements, myoclonic jerks and epileptic fits are common. Many patients have problems with vision and speech. Sometimes muscle fasciculation is seen with atrophy e.g. in the small hand muscles. Progression produces mute, rigid, immobile patients ending in coma.

The CSF is usually normal but the EEG is abnormal showing generalised repetitive discharges on a background of diffuse slow activity. There is no specific therapy.

Subacute sclerosing panencephalitis (SSPE) is a rare disease largely affecting children. Patches of sclerosis are seen in the brain accompanied by intranuclear inclusion bodies in the neurones and glial cells suggesting a viral infection. It is probably caused by the measles virus. Patients present with intellectual decline, often a failure at school. This may be accompanied by personality and behaviour changes. Later fits and myoclonic jerks appear and then physical decline with the development of rigidity, pyramidal signs, cortical blindness and mutism. The mean survival is about three years: rarely very 'damaged' patients may survive. The CSF shows an elevated gamma globulin. The EEG shows a characteristic abnormality with high voltage repetitive discharges synchronous with the myoclonic jerks. High levels of anti-measles antibodies are often found in the serum and CSF. No specific treatment is effective.

Communicating hydrocephalus (low pressure hydrocephalus) describes either a failure in the formation or in the absorption of CSF, or an obstruction to the CSF flow over the surface of the brain. In many instances the cause may be from previous trauma, meningitis or an SAH. A group of older patients may present with dilated ventricles, without intraventricular obstruction, where the CSF pressure is normal or only slightly elevated (sometimes this is paroxysmal).

In this last group the common presenting symptoms are progressive dementia, urinary incontinence and marked ataxia with the appearance of an unsteady broad-based gait with short shuffling steps. In such patients the CSF is usually normal and under normal pressure. The CT scan may show some ventricular dilatation often with absent surface cerebral sulci on the high cuts. An AEG shows air in the dilated ventricles but not over the surface, and an RIHSA scan may show the isotope passing into the ventricles where it stays without the usual rapid spread over the surface.

In selected patients a ventriculo-atrial or ventriculo-peritoneal shunt may produce improvement. However some patients do not benefit and the shunts themselves seem prone to complications, particularly the development of secondary infections, subdural haematomata, and blockage.

Multi-infarct dementia is caused by repeated small cerebral infarcts often accompanied by physical changes. In such patients there may be a history of 'strokes' or hypertension and in many, focal neurological symptoms and signs. Recognition may be aided by the use of the 'ischaemic score' (Hachinski *et al.,* 1975). Scoring is made by: abrupt onset 2, step-wise deterioration 1, fluctuating course 2, nocturnal confusion 1, relative preserved personality 1, depression 1, somatic complaints 1, emotional incontinence 1, history of hypertension 1, history of 'stroke' 2, evidence of associated atheroma 1, focal neurological symptoms 2, focal neurological signs 2. A score of more than 8/18 suggests this mechanism and many patients show scores of 10–12. A CT scan shows atrophy with multiple areas of low density (Plate 13). There is evidence of reduced cerebral blood flow and some evidence that anticoagulants may prevent deterioration.

Motor Neurone Disease

This is a degenerative disease of unknown cause which progressively destroys the motor nerve cells in the spinal cord, cortico-spinal tracts and motor nuclei of the cranial nerves. The three components, progressive muscular atrophy (anterior horn cells), amyotrophic lateral sclerosis (cortico-spinal tracts) and progressive bulbar palsy (cranial nerve nuclei) are commonly combined but some patients may show predominant involvement of one of the three. It usually presents in late middle life with a mean duration of 3–5 years: those with bulbar palsy have a shorter survival whereas some patients with predominant muscular atrophy may survive ten years or more. Rare families are described with dominant inheritance and an early onset.

The symptoms and signs are a mixture of upper and lower motor neurone involvement with muscle weakness, wasting and widespread fasciculation. These are common in the arms and hands often accompanied by exaggerated reflexes. Often the legs are stiff and spastic, but may show wasting and fasciculation. Bulbar involvement causes speech and swallowing disturbance with the appearance of a wasted fasciculating tongue. Sometimes an asymmetrical presentation causes diagnostic difficulty. Sensation and sphincter functions are spared although cramps are common. Later spinal, neck and respiratory muscles may be involved.

EMG studies will confirm widespread denervation in the limbs with preservation of motor conduction velocity (until very late). With widespread neurogenic atrophy there may be a mild rise in the CK, and the CSF protein may also be mildly elevated. In patients with bulbar symptoms myasthenia and thyrotoxicosis must be excluded.

No treatment is effective but patients and their families require considerable support with symptomatic treatment and provision of various aids.

Heredo-familial Degenerative Disorders

There are numerous rare inherited degenerative disorders affecting the CNS. One of the more common in the group of spino-cerebellar degenerations is *Friedreich's ataxia*. This is a recessive disorder, rarely dominant, causing degeneration in the posterior and lateral columns of the spinal cord and in the cerebellum.

The disease usually presents early, between the ages of 7–15 years, and slowly progresses. Many patients survive 20–30 years, often dying from cardiac involvement.

Symptoms and signs include a slowly progressive ataxia, initially affecting gait but later co-ordination in the limbs, accompanied by dysarthria and nystagmus. There may be limb weakness, particularly the legs, from cortico-spinal tract involvement, often with extensor plantar responses, although the tendon reflexes are lost from damage to the dorsal roots and posterior columns. Posterior column sensory modalities are impaired.

Many patients show skeletal abnormalities with pes cavus and a scoliosis. Optic atrophy and deafness may occur. A significant proportion of patients have myocardial involvement with conduction defects and even heart failure (the ECG is abnormal). Diabetes mellitus is common, c. 20%.

EMG studies may show slowing of conduction with impaired sensory action potentials. The CSF is usually normal.

There is no specific treatment although orthopaedic procedures may be used to help correct deformities. Physiotherapy may aid mobility.

Cerebellar degenerations are another rare group where progressive cerebellar neuronal loss is accompanied by increasing cerebellar signs. Some are familial and many have a late onset. In some patients there is more widespread involvement with pyramidal and extra-pyramidal signs and dementia. CT scanning or an AEG will show cerebellar atrophy often with an enlarged fourth ventricle.

Peroneal muscular atrophy (Charcot-Marie-Tooth disease) is dominantly inherited (rarely sporadic). It starts with weakness and wasting in the peroneal muscles (ankle evertors) and in time produces the so-called 'inverted champagne bottle' shaped leg with marked wasting from the lower third of the thigh distally. The distal arm and hand muscles may be involved causing wasting and clawing. The leg reflexes are lost and the arm reflexes depressed or absent. There may be distal sensory impairment (usually mild). Pes cavus develops early with clawed toes and later the foot may become 'flail' from weakness of the ankle plantar and dorsiflexors. The cause is neurogenic and a proportion of patients have thickened peripheral nerves.

EMGs commonly show slowed conduction velocities with reduced or absent sensory action potentials. A nerve biopsy may show features of repeated de- and remyelination. A second group of patients can be recognised with relatively normal conduction velocities and nerves that are not thickened. Here neuronal degeneration seems to be the primary pathological change.

The disease runs a very slow course with insidious progression. Treatment is ineffective. Surgical appliances, such as below knee calipers, may help mobility by producing a 'stable' ankle.

Various other types of heredo-familial degenerative neuropathy are recognised often by associated features, e.g. *Dejerine-Sottas* where the neuropathy is linked with thickened nerves and ataxia from sensory loss, and *Refsum's disease,* where excess phytanic acid in the body causes a peripheral neuropathy, cerebellar disturbance, retinal upset with night blindness, skin, skeletal and cardiac abnormalities.

16. BASAL GANGLIA DISEASE

The basal ganglia include the corpus striatum (caudate and lenticular nuclei) and associated nuclei (the red and sub-thalamic nuclei and substantia nigra). Damage or disease in these pathways causes involuntary movements which may be accompanied by changes in muscle tone and by rigidity.

Involuntary movements

Tremors are rhythmic alternating contractions which are described in several ways (Table XVI). *Chorea* describes continuous irregular involuntary movements; hemichorea is unilateral. Sometimes these movements become very forceful involving proximal muscles so the limbs wildly jerk about—hemi-ballismus (most commonly caused by a vascular lesion in the contralateral subthalamic nucleus). *Athetosis* describes an instability of posture with the appearance of writhing involuntary movements: it may merge into a more florid dystonia with sustained irregular postures produced by muscle spasm with exaggerated tone. Many of the conditions causing athetosis relate to long-standing developmental brain damage. Torsion dystonia is a rare disabling condition sometimes appearing as an inherited disorder, sometimes sporadically, and even more rarely as a symptom of

Table XVI

Tremor

Positional Tremor (best shown holding the arms outstretched)
  1. Benign essential tremor
  2. Anxiety (fine)
  3. Metabolic
      (a) thyrotoxic: fine, rapid
      (b) liver ⎫
          renal ⎭ failure: coarse, may 'flap'
      (c) Wilson's disease
      (d) alcohol, drugs e.g. lithium

Action Tremor (intention tremor worse on movement)
   Cerebellar lesions

Rest Tremor
   Parkinson's disease

Senile Tremor (both at rest and action)

other basal ganglia disease. Spasmodic torticollis is a sustained spasm of the sternomastoid muscles causing a 'wry neck'. The cause is unknown—rarely it is symptomatic but often it is considered as a functional variety of a dystonia.

Tremor

This may be a symptom of many disorders (Table XVI). The commonest cause of tremor occurring at rest is Parkinson's disease.

Positional tremor is commonly seen in patients with *benign essential tremor*. This is a dominant inherited disorder often apparent from an early age getting slowly worse with time. In addition to the arms being affected it may involve the head, jaw, lips, tongue and even the legs. It is worse under stress and may be relieved by alcohol. Simple sedatives as benzodiazepines may help and some patients are improved by the beta blocker, propranolol.

Parkinson's disease (paralysis agitans)

This is the commonest basal ganglia disorder being a degenerative condition of unknown cause affecting the nigro-striatal pathways. In a few instances it may follow encephalitis (usually lethargica) or be induced by a number of drugs, particularly phenothiazines, butyrophenones and reserpine. Similar symptoms may appear in association with certain uncommon disorders as Wilson's disease, progressive supranuclear palsy, or follow severe head injuries, manganese intoxication or carbon monoxide poisoning.

The main clinical findings are the appearance of *tremor* which is present at rest, disappearing with movement. This is described as 'pill-rolling' with a rate of 4–8 Hz. It is accompanied by rigidity which has a 'cog wheel' (broken up) feeling. If there is doubt about this change in tone it can be sometimes emphasised in the arm under test, by asking patients to open and close the opposite hand. The *rigidity* causes a flexed posture and there are associated changes with poor balance, a festinating (hurrying) walk, difficulties turning, getting out of a low chair or turning in bed. Difficulty in initiating movement is accompanied by *bradykinesia*, greatly slowed movement, which commonly results in complaints of weakness, although given time, power is usually well preserved. Patients have a mask-like impassive face, a soft slow speech and writing diminishing in size. Many patients notice blepharospasm, difficulty in opening the eyes, and may show blepharoclonus (involuntary 'clonic' fluttering of the lightly closed eye-lids) and a positive glabellar tap. Pooling of saliva with dribbling is frequent and constipation common. Many patients have poor appetite and weight loss. Although original reports stated that the 'senses and intellect' were spared, some patients complain of sensory symptoms—pain, restlessness, even 'burning', and in those with long-standing disease there may be intellectual deterioration. Depression is common.

The disease which affects older patients, tends to progress slowly so that two thirds are severely disabled or dead after ten years.

With the recognition of a number of neurotransmitters in the basal ganglia new approaches to treatment have arisen. Two are well recognised—acetylcholine (ACh) which is excitatory and dopamine which is inhibitory. Other transmitters are also involved. In Parkinson's disease the nigrostriatal content of dopamine is depleted.

Treatment: was originally with anticholinergic drugs: benzhexol, orphenadrine, benztropine, procyclidine and benapryzine are the best known. They cause moderate benefit (about 15% improvement on disability scores) but they have as side-effects confusion, blurred vision (aggravating glaucoma), dry mouth, urinary retention and constipation.

Dopamine does not cross the blood-brain barrier so cannot be used but its immediate precursor dopa (L-dihydroxyphenylalanine) does. However in order to get a reasonable dose of dopa into the CNS a very large oral dose has to be given and this often causes side-effects (largely nausea and vomiting). This is because dopa decarboxylase in the gut and tissues breaks down dopa to dopamine. To overcome this two dopa-decarboxylase inhibitors have been introduced, benserazide and alpha-methyldopahydrazine. Either of these combined with dopa allows a low dose to be given orally which reaches the CNS. These combined preparations Madopar (benserazide + dopa), and Sinemet (methyldopahydrazine + dopa) are taken after food and the dose slowly increased. The main limiting side-effect is the appearance of dyskinetic involuntary movements. Other side-effects include confusional states, nausea and vomiting, postural hypotension and rarely cardiac arrhythmias.

Although about two thirds of patients show a good response to dopa it is disappointing in about one third. Furthermore with prolonged use in many patients the benefit wears off and oscillations in daily performance are found with an 'on-off' effect.

Amantadine, originally introduced as an antiviral agent, may also produce benefit with about 15% improvement in function. The dose is low, 100 mg b.d., and there are few side-effects. It has a synergistic action with other anti-Parkinsonian drugs.

Attempts have also been made to use dopamine agonists as bromocriptine. This is expensive and high doses are often necessary. It has similar side-effects to dopa.

For strictly unilateral Parkinson's disease with severe tremor not responding well to drug therapy, there may be a place for stereotactic surgery, making a lesion in the ventrolateral nucleus of the thalamus.

Steele-Richardson-Olszewski's syndrome (progressive supranuclear palsy)

This describes a progressive neuronal degeneration affecting the basal ganglia, mid-brain, brain stem and cerebellum. Patients usually present in late middle age with a supranuclear gaze palsy, initially with lost volitional vertical eye movements and complaints of visual difficulties. These are usually accompanied by extra-pyramidal features with rigidity of the face, neck and trunk, and pyramidal and cerebellar signs. Many patients become demented, ending up rigid, bed-ridden with an almost total supranuclear paralysis of eye movements.

Wilson's disease

This is a recessive disorder producing damage in the corpus striatum and hepatic cirrhosis largely from the deposition of copper. Patients may present in childhood with features of liver failure, or with involuntary movements, particularly choreo-athetoid movements and a 'flapping' tremor, or more rarely with an akinetic-rigid syndrome. Dysarthria is usually marked and there may be a dementia and sometimes dystonia. Patients show a Kayser-Fleischer ring, a zone of golden brown pigment in the cornea near the limbus (best seen with a slit lamp) due to copper deposition.

Laboratory findings should include abnormal liver function tests, a low serum copper (< 15 μmol/l), a low caeruloplasmin (< 200 μg/l), a high urinary copper excretion (> 3.2 μmol/day) and an increased copper content in a liver biopsy (> 250 μg/g dry weight).

Treatment is with D-penicillamine (1–2 g/day). This needs to be maintained: side-effects include renal damage and thrombocytopenia.

Chorea

Sydenham's chorea (St. Vitus' dance)

This originally occurred in children or young adults in association with acute rheumatism. Patients appear clumsy, dropping objects and show typical choreic fidgets which may involve the face, limbs and trunk. They are aggravated by stress. Hypotonia is present and the arms will hyperpronate if held outstretched above the head. Attempts at maintaining a smooth strong grip fail as irregular inco-ordinate muscular contractions occur. Patients often have difficulty in protruding the tongue. In walking there may be a 'dancing' gait. The reflexes are often brisk.

Many patients show features of a rheumatic carditis (murmurs, cardiac enlargement or failure, and pericarditis) and arthritis. However the chorea may follow the infection after an interval. Evidence of a recent rheumatic infection by streptococci may be shown by a raised antistreptolysin titre, culture from a throat swab, and supported by changes in the FBC, ESR, and an abnormal ECG (particularly a prolonged PR interval). In acute form chorea is exhausting and patients need bed rest and sedation.

Chorea may also appear in *pregnancy* (chorea gravidarum) and more commonly now in women taking an oestrogen-containing oral contraceptive pill. Stopping the 'pill' allows recovery. Other drugs may induce chorea, e.g. phenytoin, and rarely it may appear in patients with polycythaemia rubra vera, SLE and thyrotoxicosis. *Huntington's chorea* (page 100) should not be forgotten.

Myoclonus

This describes brief rapid shock-like involuntary movements, jerks often synchronously involving many muscles. Such jerks may occur repetitively in the same muscles and mild degrees are common in epileptic patients, often on waking and sometimes as a prodrome to a major fit. Myoclonic jerks may also occur in a number of metabolic disturbances e.g. renal or hepatic failure, anoxia, and alcohol withdrawal. They may occur in rare degenerative cerebral disorders e.g. Jakob-Creutzfeldt's disease, SSPE, and even more rarely in progressive myoclonic epilepsy.

Clonazepam may be useful in the treatment of myoclonus; other types of anticonvulsants may also be used.

17. PERIPHERAL NEUROPATHY

In peripheral and cranial nerves there may be damage to the myelin sheath (demyelination) or to the cell body and axon resulting in degeneration. Often there is a combination of the two. Repair by remyelination is relatively

Table XVII
Causes of Peripheral Neuropathy

1. Trauma	Direct compression, chronic entrapment
2. Metabolic	B_{12} deficiency (pernicious anaemia)
	B_1 deficiency (often malabsorption)
	Diabetes mellitus
	Uraemia
	Hepatic failure
	Porphyria
	Amyloidosis
3. Poisoning	Alcohol
	Drugs—INAH, nitrofurantoin, vincristine
	Metals—Lead, gold
	Organo-phosphates—tri-orthocresyl phosphate
4. Infective	Diphtheria
	Leprosy
5. Guillain-Barré	(Often post-infective)
6. Vascular	Connective tissue disorders—rheumatoid, PAN, Diabetes
7. Carcinomatous	Entrapment—myeloma, lymphoma
	Non-metastatic
	'Cuffing' of roots by carcinoma
8. Heredo-familial	Peroneal muscular atrophy, Refsum's disease
9. Senile	

rapid but repeated episodes of demyelination followed by repair may cause thickening of nerves. Regeneration is slow (over many months) and may be incomplete.

Presentation

Symptoms and signs of a neuropathy usually start distally in the longest fibres i.e. in the feet and hands. Sensory symptoms include tingling, numbness, pain or sensations of walking on wool. These are commonly accompanied by weakness. In the feet, a 'foot-drop' may appear and progress to a 'flail' foot with weakness of the ankle plantar and dorsiflexors. As weakness spreads proximally there will be difficulty getting out of a low chair, or out of bed, or in climbing steps. In the hands fine manipulative movements may be disturbed, e.g. doing up small buttons, writing or unscrewing bottle tops. In the arms weakness may produce problems with shaving, brushing hair or lifting objects. Bulbar and facial muscle weakness may cause difficulties with speech and swallowing. Trunk, spinal, neck and respiratory muscles may also weaken. Progressive sensory loss may spread up the trunk, and even to the face. Autonomic involvement, most common in diabetics, may cause micturition and bowel upsets, impotence and loss of sweating. Postural hypotension may cause 'giddy, faint feelings' and visual blurring may arise from accommodation weakness.

With a neuropathy of some duration it is common for muscles to waste and show fasciculation. In time they may be replaced by fibrous tissue and contractures may appear. The tendon reflexes are usually depressed or absent. In mild cases only the ankle jerks may be lost. If weakness is severe in the feet no plantar response can be elicited. Sensory impairment often involves all modalities spreading from a glove-stocking distribution, with sometimes a level on the trunk. Certain sized fibres may be selectively damaged causing changing patterns; e.g. pain and temperature are largely carried by small fibres.

Most peripheral neuropathies are mixed, but in a few instances may be largely sensory or motor. Patchy involvement of several isolated peripheral nerves, e.g. an ulnar and lateral popliteal nerve, is termed a *mononeuritis multiplex*. This may be caused by: (i) leprosy, (ii) connective tissue disorders (from thrombotic endarteritis of the vasa nervorum with infarction of nerves), e.g. rheumatoid arthritis, polyarteritis nodosa, (iii) diabetes mellitus, (iv) sarcoidosis, and (v) local nerve infiltration by carcinoma or lymphoma.

With *increasing age,* many patients show signs of a mild neuropathy with absent ankle jerks, lost vibration sense in the toes and an elevated two point threshold in the finger tips. In many of these patients (aged more than 70) this is a senile degeneration, although in a few, diabetes or other causes are responsible.

Simple pressure palsies

These may cause local nerve lesions, e.g. a wrist drop from a radial nerve palsy (Saturday night palsy). These most commonly are seen in patients who have developed nerve damage from pressure occurring in a 'deep sleep' often induced by drugs or alcohol. With time most recover well.

Chronic entrapment palsies include:

1. *Median nerve compression* in the carpal tunnel at the wrist. Patients present with nocturnal tingling and pain in the fingers and hand with proximal radiation. There may be sensory impairment in the median ($3\frac{1}{2}$) fingers and wasting and weakness of abductor pollicis brevis. Often the nerve is tender at the wrist and a blood pressure cuff inflated around the arm may provoke similar symptoms. Certain medical conditions may present as a carpal tunnel

lesion—myxoedema, diabetes, acromegaly, rheumatoid arthritis, and myeloma.

2. *Ulnar nerve compression* at the elbow presents with complaints of numbness and tingling in the ulnar (1½) fingers of the hand with weakness and wasting of the ulnar innervated intrinsic hand muscles (particularly the first dorsal interosseous and abductor digiti minimi) and the long finger flexors of the ring and little finger tips and the ulnar wrist flexor. The ulnar nerve is commonly thickened at the elbow.

3. *Lateral popliteal nerve compression* occurs at the head of the fibula, usually presenting with complaints of pain, tingling and numbness over the dorsum of the foot and antero-lateral shin with a foot-drop from weakness of the ankle dorsiflexors and evertors. The ankle jerk is preserved. Occasionally a ganglion or neuroma at the head of the fibula may be responsible.

EMG studies are often diagnostic showing the site of entrapment.

Metabolic Neuropathies

Diabetes mellitus

This is the commonest cause of neuropathy seen in Great Britain. Usually it causes a *distal symmetrical neuropathy* largely involving sensation with tingling, numbness and sometimes burning in the toes and feet. Later the hands may be involved. The ankle jerks are lost and later other tendon jerks. Vibration sense in the toes is lost early, later other sensory modalities. In some patients neuropathic joints and perforating ulcers in the feet may appear.

An acute *proximal mononeuropathy* of the femoral nerve (diabetic amyotrophy) also may occur (page 92). Diabetes may produce a *mononeuritis multiplex* with patchy peripheral and cranial nerve involvement and sometimes an *autonomic neuropathy*. In the latter, impotence, episodes of nocturnal diarrhoea, postural hypotension and disordered sweating are usually the manifestations.

In many patients excellent control of the diabetes may allow a good degree of recovery but this does not always happen.

B_{12} Deficiency

This causes pernicious anaemia with a macrocytosis and megaloblastic marrow. It may also cause dementia, subacute combined degeneration in the spinal cord (with involvement of posterior and lateral columns) and optic atrophy. It most commonly causes a peripheral neuropathy with distal sensory symptoms, mild distal weakness and lost ankle jerks. The plantar responses may be extensor if there is cord involvement. Patients with cord involvement have signs of a peripheral neuropathy.

A low serum B_{12} level (< 150 pg/ml), blood film, marrow and Schilling test for B_{12} absorption will confirm the diagnosis. Treatment with injections of hydroxocobalamin, 1000 μg/day for ten days and then monthly will usually reverse the neuropathy. Cord damage may be arrested but does not always recover.

B_1 Deficiency

This may occur in patients with malabsorption or from severe malnutrition often combined with other deficiencies. It causes a distal symmetrical mixed polyneuropathy often accompanied by 'burning' feet and foot-drop. Recovery may occur after treatment with large doses of thiamine (100 mg daily) but is usually slow and not always complete. The neuropathy of chronic alcoholism may in part be due to thiamine deficiency.

Porphyria

This may present acutely with abdominal pain, an acute psychosis, epileptic fits or an acute neuropathy. The last is largely motor producing a flaccid paralysis and may affect the arms more than the legs. Proximal muscles are more often affected. The reflexes are lost early. Bulbar and facial involvement occurs frequently and there may be respiratory failure. There may be sensory disturbance and sphincter upset. In many instances an acute crisis is precipitated by vomiting, pregnancy or more commonly drugs, particularly barbiturates. All patients show a persistent tachycardia and some transient hypertension.

The diagnosis can be confirmed by the detection of porphyrins in the urine. If left to stand, urine from such patients may turn dark red. The CSF is usually normal. Inappropriate secretion of ADH may occur.

In the acute phase support in the ICU may be necessary if there is bulbar or respiratory involvement. Most patients recover slowly although a few are left with deficit. The pattern of recovery suggests the pathogenesis involves degeneration followed by regeneration.

Carcinomatous involvement

Malignant cells may locally compress peripheral or cranial nerves or 'cuff' nerve roots. This may be seen in carcinomatous meningeal infiltration which may cause multiple cranial nerve palsies.

Figures vary for the incidence of neuromyopathic involvement from a non-metastatic effect of a carcinoma remote from the nerve and values from 5–15% have been given. Recognition and removal of the carcinoma may allow recovery. The commonest sources are bronchus (small cell), breast, ovary, stomach, lymphomas and myeloma. The neuropathy is usually a distal mixed sensory-motor disturbance. Other complications are listed on page 128.

Investigations

These should include an FBC, ESR, urea, electrolytes, liver function tests, lipid profile, and serum B_{12} level. In patients suspected of B_1 deficiency a red cell transketolase should be added. In all patients blood glucose levels, fasting and after a glucose load, should be estimated. If malabsorption is suspected then calcium, folate levels and faecal fat excretion should be measured. In those suspected of connective tissue disorders auto-antibodies, ANF, RA, Latex, and DNA binding may be added. Estimates of blood lead or phytanic acid (Refsum's disease) may be indicated. Rare endocrine causes need exclusion, e.g. hypothyroidism, acromegaly.

A urine specimen should always be sent for chemical analysis and screening for porphyrins.

CSF examination is seldom diagnostic. In many patients with a neuropathy the protein may be mildly elevated. Increased cell counts, largely lymphocytic, may be found in sarcoidosis, and malignant cells may be found in patients with carcinomatous infiltration (often associated with a very low CSF glucose). X-rays of the chest should be taken.

Nerve conduction studies are important. Needle sampling of affected muscles will usually show if denervation is present, indicating axonal degeneration has occurred. Primary muscle disease can be excluded for it produces specific changes. Complete denervation will cause conduction loss. Most peripheral nerves consist of many thousands of fibres and only some of these may be damaged: conduction in the undamaged fibres may be normal. However if a proportion of nerve fibres (axons) have been damaged then the amplitude of the evoked muscle, nerve or sensory action potentials will be diminished or they will be absent. In demyelination of peripheral nerves there is usually signifcant slowing of conduction velocity. Local sites of nerve entrapment may be clearly shown, e.g. carpal tunnel.

Nerve biopsy will usually show axonal degeneration or demyelination, findings that can be obtained from conduction studies. It is only possible to get a clear diagnosis from biopsy in a few instances where a nerve may be locally infiltrated, e.g. in leprosy or amyloidosis. If the vasa nervorum have been involved, e.g. in polyarteritis, this may also be seen at biopsy.

Treatment

Treatment depends on recognition of the cause and its correction. In many instances no cause is found and many such patients are treated with a mixture of vitamins. Physiotherapy and aids, e.g. a caliper to correct a foot-drop, may be helpful. Active exercises will help recovering muscles to function more efficiently.

In a few patients where progression continues and the CSF protein is high, a course of steroids may be tried, sometimes with benefit. In many older patients the gradual onset of a progressive neuropathy may be the herald of an occult malignant process. Here follow up may give an answer if initial screening tests prove negative.

18. MUSCLE DISEASE

Myopathy describes a disorder of skeletal muscle and most patients present with muscle weakness shown by abnormalities in limb movements, gait, posture and facial expression. Weakness usually starts in proximal limb muscles. In the legs this causes difficulty in rising from lying, getting out of a low chair or bath or stepping on to a high step. Later there is walking difficulty as weakness spreads, particularly if this is combined with trunk muscle weakness, where a lordotic posture appears with a protuberant abdomen. In the arms weakness of shoulder muscles leads to difficulties in movements above the shoulders, e.g. shaving, brushing hair, putting on make-up. Facial muscle weakness may produce an immobile face lacking expression with ptosis. Difficulties in full eye closure and whistling may be early signs. Bulbar muscle weakness may cause difficulties in speech and swallowing. The neck muscles, particularly the extensors, may become weak.

With time affected muscles waste. They may be replaced by fibrous tissue with the appearance of contractures and deformities. The tendon reflexes are depressed or lost relatively late. There is no sensory loss. Sphincter function is usually spared. In some conditions cardiac and respiratory muscles may also be involved.

Although degrees of muscle weakness may be classified by MRC grades (page 12) a functional assessment based on patients' ability to perform certain tasks proves of great value in determining disability and in following progress.

Investigations

These include an FBC, ESR, urea, electrolytes, blood glucose and calcium (preferably fasting) and tests of thyroid function. Certain other endocrine studies may be indicated. In the inflammatory myopathies, tests to exclude connective tissue disorders are important. An ECG should be performed to exclude myocardial involvement. Many enzymes in the blood may be elevated when muscle is damaged, but creatine phosphokinase (CK) levels are the most useful index of active muscle disease.

An EMG is important as this will exclude neuropathic disorders and needle sampling of affected muscles will often confirm a myopathic process by the presence of short duration, low amplitude polyphasic potentials.

The most useful investigation is *biopsy* of an affected muscle. The tissue obtained should be studied histochemically as well as by routine staining for microscopy. Sections should also be prepared for electron microscopy. It is

Table XVIII
Muscle Disease

Muscular Dystrophies (inherited disorders)	
Duchenne	X-linked recessive
Limb-girdle	Recessive or sporadic
Facio-scapulo-humeral	Dominant
Ocular	Dominant
Associated with Myotonia (delay in relaxation)	
Dystrophia myotonica	Dominant
Myotonia congenita	Dominant or recessive
Inflammatory myopathies	
Polymyositis	Acute, subacute
	Associated with connective tissue disorders—malignant disease
Polymyalgia rheumatica	
Sarcoidosis	
Endocrine myopathies	
Thyrotoxic	
Hypothyroidism	
Steroid excess	Cushing's, iatrogenic
Acromegaly	
Hyperparathyroidism	
Osteomalacia	
Electrolyte disturbances	
Low potassium	Familial periodic paralysis, Conn's syndrome
Drugs	Chloroquine, beta blockers, alcohol
Metabolic disturbances	Myophosphorylase deficiency (McArdle's disease)
Carcinomatous neuromyopathies	

important that a biopsy site is chosen from a muscle that has not been subjected to needling (e.g. by EMG or injections) and which is not so severely affected as largely to consist of fibrous tissue.

Other special investigations may be indicated such as an ischaemic exercise test to estimate the normal rise in lactate values in the blood (Munzat, 1970).

Muscle diseases are classified in many ways (Table XVIII). The *muscular dystrophies* include a group of uncommon genetically determined disorders. Correct labelling is important in giving a prognosis, genetic counselling, and carrier identification, although to date no known cause has been found. The usual mode of inheritance is indicated in Table XVIII.

Muscular Dystrophies

Duchenne dystrophy

This is the most common, inherited as an X-linked recessive so that boys are affected and transmission is via their unaffected mothers who are carriers. About 80% of carriers can be detected by (i) repeated CK values (at least three), (ii) abnormal EMGs, and (iii) muscle biopsies.

Affected boys usually present by the age of two to three with frequent falls and a waddling gait. As they attempt to rise, they 'climb up' themselves using their arms to assist their weak proximal leg muscles. Tight heel cords appear early so boys appear to walk on their toes. Sometimes there are complaints of leg pains, and the calves may appear disproportionately bulky when compared with the thinner thigh muscles—termed pseudohypertrophy. As the weakness progresses a severe kyphoscoliosis develops and many boys are confined to a wheel-chair by the ages of 12–15. Further muscle involvement leads to respiratory complications, often bronchopneumonia. About 70% have abnormal ECGs (tall R waves in right precordial and deep Q waves in limb and left precordial leads). The CK is elevated, the EMG abnormal and muscle biopsy characteristic. Many boys have a lower IQ than expected. Most die late in their second or early in their third decade.

Limb-girdle dystrophy

This usually presents in early adult life but may present later. Some patients appear to have a sporadic form. The disease affects the girdles and proximal limb muscles running a very slow course. Considerable variation is seen in different families and between patients. Later in life patients may be confined to a wheel-chair and develop cardiopulmonary complications.

Facio-scapulo-humeral dystrophy

This usually presents in childhood with involvement of the facial muscles. Later as the muscles of the shoulder girdles, neck and upper arms are involved weakness becomes apparent and a typical appearance is seen. There may be involvement of leg muscles, usually proximal, but occasionally distal. Progression is slow and many patients have a normal life span although disabled.

Ocular myopathy

This presents with bilateral ptosis. Later a progressive ophthalmoplegia develops causing marked loss of eye movements in all directions. There are seldom complaints of diplopia. There may be facial muscle weakness and in some patients bulbar upset with dysphagia. Rarely proximal limb muscles may be affected. Progression is slow and most patients have a normal life span.

Dystrophia myotonica

This is dominantly inherited and patients show a number of characteristic defects in addition to the muscular disorder. Typically the symptoms start in adolescence with a myopathic face, delayed relaxation in finger grip ('sticky fingers') and distal weakness in the feet and hand muscles. The neck muscles are commonly affected and weakness spreads proximally in the limbs and into the bulbar muscles. Many patients have cataracts, premature frontal balding, myocardial involvement and often multiple endocrine abnormalities. Many patients die prematurely from cardiopulmonary failure. Some 70% have abnormal ECGs, largely conduction defects.

The disease may appear in infancy where usually the weak facial and bulbar muscles cause feeding difficulties. The muscles appear hypotonic and motor milestones are delayed.

Myotonia congenita (Thomsen's disease)

This may have a dominant or recessive inheritance. Patients are not weak, but most complain of stiffness on starting movement. With continued exercise this improves although exposure to cold may aggravate the stiffness. EMG studies are characteristic.

Myotonia may be helped by a variety of drugs—procainamide, phenytoin or prednisolone. These do not help the muscle weakness in myotonia dystrophica.

Inflammatory Myopathies

Polymyositis

This is an acquired inflammatory disorder usually running an acute or subacute course. Often there is skin involvement, dermatomyositis. The disease may be associated with connective tissue disorders (25% rheumatoid arthritis, SLE or systemic sclerosis) and, particularly in older male patients, with an occult carcinoma.

If there is skin involvement a blotchy flush appears over the face, neck and often the hands. The onset of weakness may be very acute with involvement of proximal limb muscles: often trunk, neck and bulbar muscles are affected. Pain and muscle tenderness only appear in about 50% but about 33% describe rheumatic symptoms and about 33% Raynaud's phenomenon. About 35% of patients show atrophy of muscles and contractures. The disease may run a very variable course—acute deterioration, relapses and remissions or a chronic grumbling form.

The CK is usually very high and the ESR often elevated. EMG studies show myopathic changes but sometimes fibrillation, and the biopsy is characteristic with inflammatory cellular infiltration in the muscle. About 30% show an abnormal ECG and the vital capacity may be depressed. However in some patients tests may prove normal: the ESR in 45%, the CK in 33%, the EMG in 18% and the biopsy in 17%. Tests for connective tissue disorders and screening for an occult carcinoma may be necessary.

Treatment is usually with steroids unless there is an underlying carcinoma. In adults prednisolone 60–80 mg/day (children 1–2 mg/kg/day) is used initially and the dose titrated against patients' clinical state and CK values. Alternate day steroids may avoid some side-effects. Azathioprine may be used. Physiotherapy is important. Some two thirds of patients show a good response to treatment although some relapse as this is discontinued.

Polymyalgia rheumatica

This causes muscle pain and stiffness in elderly patients ($>$ age 60) with symptoms worse on waking and easing with use. The neck and shoulder muscles are most commonly affected. The incidence in women is double that for men. There is often associated malaise, night sweats and sometimes fever.

There is a high incidence of giant cell arteritis. It is also associated with rheumatoid arthritis, myeloma and malignant disease. The only abnormal test is the ESR which is usually very high ($>$ 70 mm/hr). The response to a low dose of steroids is dramatic. Prednisolone 20–30 mg/day should be given initially, reducing to levels of 5–10 mg/day fairly rapidly. This low dose is maintained for at least 12 months.

Endocrine Myopathies

Most patients with *thyrotoxicosis* show features of a myopathy largely affecting proximal muscles. This may be the presenting symptom. Rarely bulbar muscles may be involved and the condition may present in this way. A common complication of thyrotoxicosis is an *exophthalmic ophthalmoplegia* with limitation of upgaze. This may be associated with lid retraction and congestive vascular changes over the lateral recti. Less commonly the lateral recti may be weak. The exophthalmos pushes the eye-ball forwards.

Cushing's disease may present with proximal muscle weakness. Similar symptoms may be produced by the use of steroids (particularly the 9-alpha fluorinated compounds).

Neuromuscular Disorders

Myasthenia gravis

This causes increased fatiguability in muscle producing weakness from a defect in neuromuscular transmission. Commonly it causes fluctuating weakness so the symptoms may be missed and patients even dismissed as hysterics. It can affect all ages but most commonly affects young women. It may appear in very young children.

Common presenting features include ptosis and diplopia, facial weakness and bulbar difficulties—all often worse at the end of the day. Neck and proximal limb muscles (particularly the triceps) are usually involved. There may be respiratory and trunk muscle weakness. Intercurrent infections may precipitate acute weakness, and certain drugs, e.g. streptomycin, may make weakness worse.

Examination may show no abnormality but with exercise or prolonged muscle activity, e.g. sustained upgaze, weakness may appear. Commonly patients show ptosis, with a varying ophthalmoplegia and weakness of eye-lid closure. In more severely affected patients weakness is prominent, the vital capacity reduced and in about 15% there may be actual muscle wasting. In a few patients a purely ocular form may be present.

There is an association with thyroid disorders, connective tissue disease, pernicious anaemia and red cell aplasia. A humoral factor is suggested in the appearance of a transient form of myasthenia in neonates delivered from myasthenic mothers. Pathological changes may be found in the thymus gland: in 75% of patients this may be a lymphoid hyperplasia of the cortex and large germinal centres in the medulla. In c. 15–20% there may be a thymoma, a locally invasive tumour. Recent work has shown that the end-plates at the neuromuscular junction are morphologically abnormal and in most patients it is possible to demonstrate a raised titre of anti-acetylcholine receptor antibody in the serum (which may not be present in the purely ocular form). These findings support the view that myasthenia has an immune basis.

Diagnosis: usually clinical, supported by an edrophonium (Tensilon) test. 1–2 mg of edrophonium is injected IV and its effect followed. It is important to choose a suitable weak muscle in which improvement can be well demonstrated. If no upset occurs, the remaining 8 mg is then injected. If there is myasthenic weakness, the edrophonium will produce temporary improvement. The injection may produce transient nausea, lachrymation, and muscle flickering particularly around the eyes. Occasionally a longer lasting therapeutic trial with pyridostigmine may be necessary.

Antibodies to anti-acetylcholine receptor are usually found in patients with generalised myasthenia. Nearly 50% of patients also show antibodies to skeletal muscle and if a thymoma is present nearly all patients have muscle antibodies.

EMG studies with repetitive stimulation and measurement of muscle action potential amplitude before and after exercise may prove valuable. Single fibre studies showing the presence of neuromuscular block in fibres innervated by the same motor unit gives a higher diagnostic yield.

A chest X-ray, with lateral tomograms of the anterior mediastinum, may show the presence of a thymoma.

Other tests are occasionally used, e.g. patients with myasthenia are unusually resistant to the effect of decamethonium. Such tests should only be done in centres used to such procedures where ICU facilities are available as rarely they may provoke respiratory failure. A 'regional curare' test is sometimes used. This shows that myasthenic muscle is unduly susceptible to curare (Horowitz *et al.*, 1976).

Treatment: based on the use of anticholinesterase drugs which by blocking the break down of ACh produce increased muscle strength. However excess dosage may cause a depolarising (cholinergic) block with increased weakness. Pyridostigmine is now the drug of choice. It is given orally and the dose slowly increased to produce appropriate benefit (adult doses of 60–120 mg four to six hourly may be necessary). Neostigmine may also be used but has a more irregular absorption although it can be given by IM injection (15 mg of neostigmine orally is equivalent to 1 mg IM). Because of cholinergic side-effects, particularly diarrhoea, it may be necessary to add atropine to counter these. Details of management of bulbar and respiratory muscle weakness are given in Chapter 6.

Some patients on treatment suddenly develop increased weakness and it is important to determine if this is due to underdosage (myasthenic crisis) or overdosage (cholinergic crisis). Here a test of edrophonium may help (page 42). If patients are underdosed there is improvement, if overdosed deterioration.

Removal of the thymus gland has been shown effective as treatment with a stable remission in over 50% of patients. A further proportion of patients may be improved. Often the benefits of such surgery slowly appear over several years. There is much support for early thymectomy. If a thymoma is present, surgery is indicated. Thymectomy should be undertaken in units where an ICU is available and there is expertise in the care of such patients in the post-operative period.

With the increasing recognition of the immune basis for the disease immunosuppression with steroids and azathioprine has been tried. With steroids over two thirds of patients are improved. However in some patients on starting steroids there is an initial temporary deterioration which may be so severe that patients need intubation and assisted respiration. All patients starting steroids should be admitted to hospital. By introducing prednisolone slowly in a dose of 25 mg on alternate days, which is then increased by 5–10 mg each week to a total of 100–120 mg on alternate days, many patients do not show an initial deterioration. However most patients relapse after a few months if the steroids are discontinued. Often the steroid dose can be slowly reduced with continuing benefit.

The demonstration of anti-acetylcholine receptor antibody has allowed a new method of treatment by plasma exchange. This appears to remove the antibody and if it is combined with immunosuppressive therapy (steroids on alternate days and azathioprine 2.5 mg/kg/day) may hold patients in remission. Patients receiving immunosuppressive treatment require regular blood counts.

19. NEUROLOGICAL MANIFESTATIONS OF SOME MEDICAL DISORDERS

Many diseases may present with neurological complications. Such conditions include metabolic disorders leading to deficiency states, rare inborn errors of metabolism (e.g. porphyria, Wilson's disease), endocrine disturbances, renal or hepatic failure, electrolyte upsets and connective tissue disorders.

Malabsorption and Deficiency States

These may cause multiple deficits accompanied by marked weight loss, loss of muscle bulk and weakness. Certain vitamin deficiencies may cause specific neurological symptoms: B_{12} deficiency has been discussed (page 111).

Thiamine (B_1) deficiency may cause neurological upset. The commonest manifestation being a peripheral neuropathy. This may be associated with cardiac failure (wet beri beri). Nicotinic acid and riboflavin deficiency may also cause 'burning feet' with a neuropathy and sometimes mental changes. Alcoholics may show a similar neuropathy.

An *encephalopathy (Wernicke-Korsakoff syndrome)* may also arise from thiamine deficiency. This causes patchy small haemorrhages in the upper brain stem and hypothalamus. Patients usually present with a confusional state and deteriorating conscious level. Loss of recent memory is marked and may be accompanied by confabulation. Vomiting is common, and there may be vertigo. There are often ocular symptoms and signs: these include nystagmus (85%), a lateral rectus (54%) or conjugate gaze (44%) palsy. Ataxia is usual and many patients also have signs of a peripheral neuropathy. Although chronic alcoholism is the commonest cause it may also occur with severe malnutrition.

Thiamine deficiency may be confirmed by a low red cell transketolase level or a high pyruvate level. *Treatment* is by large doses of thiamine (initially 50–100 mg IV) which are continued until patients take a normal diet. The earlier treatment starts the more likely is recovery but a proportion have residual damage.

Folate deficiency may cause neurological upset, particularly mental changes and a peripheral neuropathy. It most commonly occurs with malabsorption. The serum and red cell folate levels are low. Treatment with folic acid will reverse the features but it is important to exclude B_{12} deficiency for folate therapy here will aggravate neurological disturbance.

Alcoholism

Acute intoxication may cause coma but more commonly chronic habituation causes neurological problems. These include *Wernicke's encephalopathy*, a *peripheral neuropathy*, a *cerebellar degeneration* and *dementia*. It may also cause a proximal myopathy.

Sudden abstinence in chronic alcoholics may lead to *withdrawal states*. These are often precipitated by injury, acute infection or a gastro-intestinal bleed. Initially there may be a period of restless agitation with tremor, sometimes accompanied by confusion. Within the first 48 hours there may be withdrawal fits. *Delirium tremens* may occur within 72 hours with acute confusion accompanied by visual hallucinations. Patients appear terrified and show a marked tremor, and overactive circulation. There is some mortality but most patients recover within four to five days. Management involves rehydration, parenteral vitamins, treatment of any precipitating cause, control of fits, and usually sedation with phenothiazines or benzodiazepines.

Endocrine disorders

Some have already been discussed—pituitary disturbances, diabetic neuropathy and thyrotoxicosis.

Adrenal deficiency may present with marked weakness, hypotension, asthenia or collapse. Plasma cortisol levels are low (< 170 nmol/l), the sodium low, the potassium raised and urea often raised. Steroid replacement is life-saving.

Excess adrenocorticoids may present as Cushing's syndrome. In addition to the usual features (page 81), a proximal myopathy and mental disturbances are common. Many patients show an elevated plasma cortisol level which remains high throughout 24 hours. Steroid excess may also follow therapy and rarely from tumours producing ACTH.

Pheochromocytomas produce excess catecholamines. These may cause paroxysmal headaches, often associated with apprehension, palpitations, sweating, pallor, nausea and vomiting. These symptoms are usually accompanied by hypertension; this may be paroxysmal or even sustained. Urinary excretion levels of vanillylmandelic acid (VMA) will be elevated, but many drugs may cause falsely raised levels. Surgical removal of secreting tumours is the treatment.

Diabetes mellitus may present with coma or a deteriorating conscious level (page 33). Many insulin treated diabetics may develop hypoglycaemic symptoms: rarely these may arise from an insulinoma.

Hepatic failure

This may arise from many different causes and present with cerebral symptoms. In patients with chronic liver disease, an acute onset of encephalopathy may be triggered by a gastro-intestinal bleed, acute infections or administration of certain drugs or alcohol. It is probable that toxic nitrogen containing materials which are normally detoxified in the liver, are shunted into the systemic circulation. The encephalopathy may cause a deteriorating conscious level or coma. There may be mental changes, confusion, fluctuating drowsiness, and alterations in mood and behaviour. Speech is often slurred and there may be a flapping tremor of the outstretched hands. Patients may show difficulties in constructional tasks and in writing. Pyramidal and extra-pyramidal signs may appear and these may even be focal. Rarely a spastic paraparesis and even a peripheral neuropathy may appear.

Many patients may have a haemorrhagic tendency with a prolonged prothrombin time. Electrolyte disturbances and severe hypoglycaemia may occur.

In many patients there is a relevant past history of liver disease with signs of liver failure as jaundice, ascites, skin stigmata and fetor. Liver function tests will be abnormal and there may be an elevated plasma ammonia in the acute encephalopathic state. The EEG will show a diffuse slow wave abnormality often with triphasic delta waves.

Treatment: by reducing protein intake, giving a high calorie sugar preparation IV and by reducing the bowel flora. Dopa and bromocriptine may produce temporary improvement.

Renal failure

This causes uraemia and may present with neurological disturbance. Chronic renal failure may cause a peripheral neuropathy, usually starting as a sensory upset in the extremities. Conduction studies show significant slowing although the pathogenesis is mixed with axonal degeneration and demyelination. It most commonly occurs in patients on dialysis and may remit after successful renal transplantation. There is also a rare encephalopathy presenting with dementia, dysarthria and fits which occurs in patients on long-term haemodialysis. With increasing uraemia, patients will show a deteriorating conscious level, confusion, coarse tremors, muscular twitching and even fits.

Electrolyte disturbances

Water intoxication with hyponatraemia may cause confusion and a deteriorating conscious level leading to coma and fits. Such patients have a low serum sodium (< 120 mmol/l). This is often due to the inappropriate secretion of antidiuretic hormone (ADH) as a complication of a number of conditions such as SAH, meningitis, polyneuritis, as a non-metastatic complication of a carcinoma (commonly bronchial) or with drugs (e.g. carbamazepine). Patients will show a low plasma osmolality (< 270 mosmol/kg) with a urine osmolality higher than that of the plasma. Recognition of the cause and fluid restriction to an intake of 500–1000 ml daily may reverse the state.

Hypokalaemia with serum potassium values < 3 mmol/l may cause marked muscle weakness. This may affect the bowel, even producing ileus, and cardiac muscle with conduction defects (causing ECG changes). The causes are most commonly potassium loss from diuretics, diarrhoea and vomiting, *Cushing's syndrome* and *hyperaldosteronism (Conn's syndrome)*. In the last, potassium loss may be so severe that patients present with episodes of profound weakness.

Familial periodic paralysis causes attacks of flaccid weakness in voluntary muscles lasting for some hours usually caused by a fall in the serum potassium. The attacks may appear on waking, after a rest or heavy meal. Spironolactone may prevent attacks.

Disturbances of calcium metabolism

Hypocalcaemia with serum concentrations of < 2 mmol/l may cause fits of varying pattern, tetany, muscle weakness and neuromuscular excitability (positive Chvostek's and Trousseau's signs) and even bulbar muscle upset. Mental changes with hallucinations, anxiety and stupor have been described. Papilloedema and cataracts may occur. Common causes are parathyroid loss (post-thyroidectomy), malabsorption and vitamin D deficiency. Diagnosis is by estimation of the serum calcium and in an acute attack IV calcium gluconate, 10–20 ml of a 10% solution, may be given with benefit.

Hypercalcaemia is often asymptomatic but with raised serum levels (> 2.6 mmol/l) patients may present with mental disturbances—often confusion, with memory impairment, depression, hallucinations or even a deteriorating conscious level. This may be associated with nausea and vomiting. There may be muscle weakness with exaggerated reflexes. Renal stones are common and many patients have polyuria and bone pains. Common causes include hyperparathyroidism, excess vitamin D intake, malignant disease, sarcoidosis and thyrotoxicosis. Diagnosis will be confirmed by a high serum calcium and the level can be lowered acutely by a saline diuresis together with frusemide and the use of steroids.

Connective tissue disorders

These include polymyalgia rheumatica (page 118), polymyositis (page 118), rheumatoid arthritis (RhA), systemic lupus erythematosus (SLE) and polyarteritis nodosa (PAN). In the last three, there may be a vasculitis leading to a thrombotic endarteritis of the vasa nervorum causing a mononeuritis multiplex.

Rheumatoid arthritis will also cause entrapment neuropathies particularly near diseased joints, a progressive sensory-motor neuropathy and a digital sensory neuropathy. It may also cause atlanto-axial subluxation with high cervical cord compression which may be life-threatening. Penicillamine treatment in patients with RhA rarely may produce a myasthenic syndrome which reverses if treatment is discontinued. Secondary amyloidosis may develop in a few patients with RhA causing a neuropathy.

Rheumatoid factor is often positive; antinuclear factor (ANF) may be normal but 40% of patients show a low titre. Anaemia and a high ESR are common.

Systemic lupus erythematosus may involve the brain and spinal cord. In the former mental disturbances, fits, pyramidal signs, ataxia, chorea and cranial nerve palsies may appear. With prolonged disease, CNS complications play an increasing part often becoming irreversible. Cord involvement with a paraparesis and a peripheral neuropathy rarely may occur.

Patients often have a positive rheumatoid factor, show hyperglobulinaemia, an elevated ESR and significant rise in DNA binding. LE cells may be detected in the peripheral blood. Some patients with SLE may show false positive tests for syphilis.

Polyarteritis nodosa causes an intense peri-arterial inflammation leading to thrombosis and infarction. This may occur in many tissues including muscle, nerve and the brain. In many patients there is malaise, weight loss, fever and often complaints of muscle pains, tenderness and wasting. Some 50–60% show a polyneuropathy, predominantly motor. Cranial nerve, brain stem, pyramidal tract and ocular lesions are relatively common. There is a high incidence of hypertension and retinopathy. Many patients also show skin changes and cardiac involvement.

Microscopic haematuria and proteinuria occur frequently. The ESR is often raised, there is hyperglobulinaemia, eosinophilia and a positive ANF in a significant proportion. Diagnosis is best established by biopsy: often an affected muscle or nerve will show typical changes in the small arteries.

Treatment: many of these conditions require steroids sometimes combined with immunosuppression. RhA is treated in many ways, largely directed towards control of joint pain, reduction of inflammation and restoring mobility.

Wegener's granuloma

This describes an aggressive invasive granuloma accompanied by a necrotising vasculitis involving midline facial structures in association with the upper respiratory tract. There is probably some overlap with PAN. The granulomata usually invade the sinuses (particularly paranasal) and nasopharynx. Involvement of the orbit is common often with a painful proptosis and ophthalmoplegia. Other tissues including the lungs, kidneys, skin, joints and heart may be involved. Some 20–50% have neurological signs, usually cranial nerve involvement, evidence of a mononeuritis multiplex or even intracranial granulomata.

Most patients have a raised ESR and anaemia. ANF tests are usually negative. Diagnosis is by biopsy. Before treatment many patients died within 12 months, however there is a good response to steroids and azathioprine.

Sarcoidosis

This produces a granulomatous or cellular infiltration characterised by endothelioid, plasma and giant cells and lymphocytes. The cause is unknown. In 7–15% there may be neurological involvement and sometimes this is the presentation although more commonly chest signs (82%), ocular signs (58%—particularly uveitis) and skin eruptions (29%—often erythema nodosum) occur. In the nervous system sarcoidosis may cause a peripheral neuropathy, often a mononeuritis multiplex, or cranial nerve palsies, the most common being a facial palsy which may be bilateral. It may also cause a meningo-encephalitis which may produce adhesions. Rarely granulomatous masses will present as hemisphere lesions or with pituitary or hypothalamic upset. Spinal cord involvement may cause a paraparesis, and a myopathy may occur.

Investigations often reveal a number of suggestive features. Over 80% show hilar gland enlargement on chest X-ray, and the Mantoux is negative in 66%. The ESR may be moderately elevated or normal. Occasionally the serum calcium is elevated. The CSF in patients with neurological involvement often shows a lymphocytic pleocytosis with elevated protein. The glucose may be normal or slightly depressed. A Kveim test is usually positive; the site should be biopsied. Lymph gland or liver biopsy may also give the diagnosis.

The course is usually slow with relapses and remissions. Some patients are helped by steroid treatment.

Neurological Syndromes Associated with Non-metastatic Malignancy

These occur in a small proportion of patients with carcinoma (most commonly bronchial) and with lymphoma.

Neuropathy

1. Peripheral sensory-motor neuropathy
2. Primary sensory neuropathy (affects dorsal roots)
3. Motor neurone disease } both very rare
4. Autonomic neuropathy }

Myopathy

1. Malignant cachexia
2. Polymyositis and dermatomyositis
3. Myopathic-myasthenic (Eaton-Lambert) syndrome
4. Myopathy caused by ectopic hormone production, e.g. ACTH

Cerebellar

A subacute progressive degeneration

Progressive multifocal leuco-encephalopathy

Foci of demyelination appear in the white matter of the hemispheres and occasionally the brain stem. It occurs most commonly in lymphomas and leukaemias and has been shown due to infection by a polyoma virus.

20. HEAD INJURIES

Most patients with acute closed head injuries causing loss of consciousness or amnesia are admitted to hospital for observation. Those with skull fractures should also be admitted. Such admissions are usually to casualty, surgical or orthopaedic wards. Patients may then be referred to a neurosurgical unit. Indications for such referral include a deteriorating conscious level, the development of focal signs, or the failure to improve as expected. Patients with obvious depressed skull fractures, compound head injuries, a persistent CSF leak, recurrent meningitis, or those suspected of certain intracranial complications, particularly expanding haematomata, will also be referred—the last may require urgent transfer.

In most closed head injuries the duration of *post-traumatic amnesia (PTA)* is a valuable guide to the severity. A duration of PTA of $<$ 24 hours indicates a moderate head injury, one to seven days a severe head injury, and more than seven days a very severe injury. In many patients there is also retrograde amnesia dating back to before the injury so that patients can give no account of the incident. This is usually of short duration (minutes).

Management

The management of all acute head injuries in which there has been loss of consciousness, amnesia or skull fracture lies in accurate serial observations to monitor progress. These include a regular assessment of conscious level (page 4), recording eye opening, best verbal and motor responses, with the pupillary reactions, respiration, pulse, BP and temperature. Fluid balance charts should also be kept. These allow any deterioration to be detected and treated.

Examination should include a careful inspection of the scalp for wounds. Bruising and swelling around the eyes are common and may prevent lid opening. However it is important to assess any optic or oculomotor nerve damage. Fractures through the skull base may cause bleeding from the ear or the appearance of blood behind the drum. Conscious patients may complain of deafness. Many patients have suffered extensive injuries which may involve the chest, abdomen and limbs which may require appropriate treatment. Some patients with significant head injuries also have neck injuries which may include a fracture-dislocation of the cervical spine. The presence of a skull fracture increases the risk of intracranial haematomata.

Clinical deterioration may be due to a number of causes. The most important to exclude immediately is an obstructed airway. Others include an expanding intracranial haematoma either from arterial or venous bleeding, the development of cerebral oedema, secondary infections, fits and less commonly severe brain damage. Such deterioration necessitates discussion with the neurosurgical team and a CT scan (if available); if meningitis could be responsible then the CSF may need examination. Skull fractures extending into the frontal or mastoid sinuses or penetrating wounds are more liable to develop infection.

On the ward head-injured patients require careful nursing. If their conscious level is depressed patients require regular charted observations, protection of the airway, positioning and regular turning. Those with absent or depressed cough and 'gag' reflexes will need regular suction, often an oral airway and sometimes intubation. In 'unconscious' patients nutrition can be maintained by nasogastric tube feeds. Such patients may need catheterisation or urinary condom drainage.

As patients recover consciousness there may be a phase of troublesome cerebral irritation when they become intermittently noisy, irritable, restless and even aggressive. Such patients are difficult to nurse but should not be heavily sedated. Most improve quickly and usually have amnesia for this period.

Overhydration, inappropriate secretion of ADH and even diabetes insipidus may occur after head injuries. Careful fluid balance charts with electrolyte and osmolality estimations aid detection and correction.

Acute Haematoma Formation

These may be extradural, subdural or intracerebral haematomata and usually present with:

1. General features of raised intracranial pressure (page 77)
2. Progressive focal neurological signs e.g. hemiparesis
3. Signs of cerebral distortion e.g. from a tentorial or foraminal pressure cone (page 78). With tentorial cones there are usually pupillary changes, third and sixth nerve involvement and then features of decerebrate rigidity. With foraminal cones a stiff neck and pyramidal signs may be accompanied by cerebellar signs and then the ominous signs of respiratory disturbance.

Patients who deteriorate or fail to improve should always be investigated further. In all patients with head injuries good quality skull X-rays should be taken. These may show fractures or displacement of a calcified pineal. A CT brain scan is the further investigation of choice. It will show any intracranial haematoma indicating its site and size. Occasionally bilateral subdural haematomata may appear isodense making recognition difficult.

Extradural haematoma

This arises from a torn arterial branch, usually the middle meningeal. The haematoma expands commonly in the temporal region, although may involve other sites. In 80% a skull fracture is present but in children the trauma may seem trivial. Presentation is usually with:
1. A deteriorating conscious level. About 33% have a lucid interval between the injury and the deterioration, the others present with a depressed conscious level.
2. Restlessness with increasing headache.
3. Increasing focal neurological signs often accompanied by a dilating pupil and slowing pulse. Some patients show a 'boggy' swelling in the temporal fossa.

Treatment is by urgent evacuation. Delay increases the mortality and morbidity. Immediate burr holes may be made if investigation or transfer involve long delays.

Subdural haematoma

This arises from torn veins connecting the cortex to the sinuses. It can be acute, presenting like an extradural or subacute presenting within 14 days of injury. It may be chronic: this is more common in the elderly with atrophic shrunken brains. About one third are bilateral. It may present insidiously with fluctuating physical and mental symptoms accompanied by headache. Signs may be focal, those of raised ICP, and often include lost upgaze and ptosis (page 72).

Treatment is surgical with evacuation through burr holes if the haematoma is of sufficient size to cause shifts or compression.

Intracerebral haematoma

This usually arises in a brain that has sustained severe traumatic damage. Many patients have been in deep coma, or have shown signs of decerebrate rigidity immediately after the injury. In the brain stem, haemorrhage may follow a transtentorial cone. Focal signs may be present. The increasing use of CT scans have shown these to be common although many sites seem clinically silent in these severely damaged brains.

Treatment by surgical evacuation has proved disappointing except in the rare cerebellar haematomata.

Cerebral oedema may develop after a head injury. Some of the brain swelling may be due to venous congestion which is directly aggravated by any respiratory obstruction or underventilation which causes CO_2 retention. A clear airway is essential. Attempts to reduce brain oedema have been made using:

1. Osmotic diuretics (page 84).
2. Steroids (dexamethasone—page 85). However their role in head injuries is debatable.
3. Controlled ventilation and hyperventilation. This may help certain patients but requires intubation and ICU facilities.

Sequelae

Many patients make a good recovery but some are left with permanent deficits, often indicating areas of damage where neuronal loss may have followed shearing of nerve fibres, actual laceration or contusion of the brain, or areas of haemorrhagic necrosis.

Permanent deficits include cranial nerve damage, particularly anosmia, blindness or visual field loss, deafness, and double vision. A hemiparesis may persist and mid-brain damage may leave unsteadiness, dysarthria and tremor. A significant proportion of patients show permanent impairment of memory, loss of higher intellectual functions, and altered behaviour and personality. These may prove major handicaps.

Epilepsy is commoner after more severe head injuries and the risks in non-missile injuries increase with the presence of a depressed skull fracture, dural tear, intracerebral haematoma or PTA > 24 hours. Some patients develop fits within the first week after an injury; this causes an increased risk of developing later fits (c. 25%). The incidence of later fits is also increased by the presence of a depressed skull fracture or acute intracerebral haematoma. Missile or penetrating brain injuries have a much higher risk of the development of fits (c. 45%), and this risk increases further if infection with abscess formation occurs. In high risk patients anticonvulsants should be prescribed.

A *persistent CSF leak* may follow injury allowing recurrent attacks of meningitis. CSF may be identified in the nose or ear by its glucose content which will react with Dextrostix whereas catarrh does not. Many CSF leaks close spontaneously but if they do not it may be necessary to close the defect surgically. Patients with a recognised CSF leak after a head injury should receive prophylactic antibiotics.

Medico-legal aspects

Junior hospital doctors may be asked to prepare medical reports or attend court to give evidence about injuries patients have received in accidents. The value of full and accurate notes made at the time of the initial examination becomes apparent. Failure to record the visual acuity, hearing or sense of smell at the initial examination on conscious patients is a common mistake.

Many patients may have amnesia at a time when they appear conscious: however at this time more complex questions will show impairment of their higher functions. It is helpful in all head-injured patients to record in their notes at the time of their discharge the duration of amnesia and any persisting defects.

In preparing reports remember that patients' permission should have been obtained and that the reports may be read by non-medical people so the language should not be over technical.

Post-concussive syndrome

Following a head injury, usually with loss of consciousness or amnesia, patients may complain bitterly of headache, dizziness, impaired concentration, blurred vision and fatigue. Often such symptoms appear aggravated by exercise. Patients may admit to irritability, depression and impaired libido or potency. Many of these symptoms have an organic basis. Cerebral contusion may cause some traumatic bleeding with meningeal irritation and headache. Sophisticated balance tests and ENG studies may show deranged brain stem and vestibular function after head injuries and in patients with amnesia of greater than 24 hours duration some impairment is commonly found on psychometric testing.

Overall such symptoms usually settle with time but adequate initial rest with reassurance and simple analgesics may be necessary. If depression becomes marked this may need treatment.

However, in many patients with only brief loss of consciousness or amnesia, the symptoms seem disproportionately severe and last a very long time. In many such patients there may be continuing litigation with a compensation issue which compounds the problem. This is sometimes called 'accident neurosis'.

In certain patients a CT scan may be necessary to exclude a chronic subdural haematoma, and formal psychometric testing may help to assess reported intellectual deficits. Where possible relatives should always be interviewed to discuss any changes in behaviour or personality. In handicapped patients, functional assessments of their daily tasks and their degree of dependence may prove most useful.

NORMAL VALUES

Haematology

Haemoglobin	M 15.5 ± 2.5 g/dl	RBC 5.5 ± 1.0 × 10^{12}/l
	F 14.0 ± 2.5 g/dl	4.8 ± 1.0 × 10^{12}/l
MCHC	32–36 g/dl	
MCH	29.5 ± 2.5 pg	
MCV	85 ± 8 fl	
PCV	M 0.40–0.54 l/l	
	F 0.35–0.47 l/l	
White cells	4.0–11.0 × 10^9/l	
Neutrophils	2.0–7.5	
Lymphocytes	1.5–4.0	
Monocytes	0.2–0.8	
Eosinophils	0.04–0.44	
Basophils	0.1	
Platelets	150–400 × 10^9/l	
Reticulocytes	0.2–2.0%	
Serum B_{12}	160–925 ng/l	
Serum folate	3–20 µg/l	
Rbc folate	160–640 µg/l	
ESR Westergren	M 0–5 mm/h	
	F 0–7 mm/h	
Wintrobe	M 0–9 mm/h	
	F 0–20 mm/h	

Slight variation occurs in different hospitals

Biochemistry

Acid phosphatase	< 5 iu/l
Alkaline phosphatase	20–100 iu/l*
Aspartate transaminase (AST)	10–50 iu/l
Bicarbonate	23–29 mmol/l
Bilirubin	3–20 µmol/l
Caeruloplasmin	300–600 µg/l
Calcium	2.2–2.7 mmol/l
Copper	13–25 µmol/l
Chloride	96–106 mmol/l
Cholesterol	3–7 mmol/l**
Creatine phosphokinase (CK)	< 50 iu/l***
Gamma-glutamyl transpeptidase (γGT)	< 50 iu/l (M), < 30 iu/l (F)
Glucose	2.8–5 mmol/l
Iron	15–35 µmol/l
TIBC	45–70 µmol/l
Lead	0.5–1.9 µmol/l
Osmolality	280–295 mosmol/kg
Phosphate	0.8–1.5 mmol/l
Potassium	3.5–5 mmol/l

Proteins	60–80 g/l
Albumin	35–45 g/l
C3	0.81–1.32 g/l
Fibrinogen	2–4 g/l
IgA	0.9–4.5 g/l
IgG	9.5–16.5 g/l
IgM	0.6–2 g/l
Sodium	130–145 mmol/l
Transketolase (red cell)	35–90 iu/l
+ thiamine pyrophosphate	4.5–40.5 %
Triglycerides	0.3–1.7 mmol/l**
Urea	2.5–7 mmol/l
Uric acid	0.1–0.4 mmol/l

* elevated in children   ** rises with age   *** varies with the laboratory

Endocrine values

Thyroid
Tri-iodothyronine (T3)	1–3 nmol/l
Total thyroxine (T4)	50–150 nmol/l
Thyroid stimulating hormone (TSH)	0–4 mu/l

Pituitary
Adrenocorticotrophic hormone (ACTH)	10–80 pg/ml
Growth hormone (GH)	< 5 ng/ml (< 10 mu/l)
Prolactin	0–5 µg/l (< 25 ng/ml)
in pregnancy	< 200 µg/l
oversecretion	> 300 ng/ml
Testosterone	3–11 nmol/l

Adrenal
Plasma cortisol
a.m.	170–720 nmol/l
Midnight	< 220 nmol/l
6 p.m.	< 400 nmol/l

FSH (Follicle Stimulating Hormone), LH (Luteinising Hormone) and Oestradiol have values that vary with the phase of the menstrual cycle.

Cerebrospinal fluid

Cells	less than 5 lymphocytes/mm³
Protein	0.2–0.45 g/l
Glucose	2.5–4.4 mmol/l (c. 60% of blood glucose level)
Lactate	< 2.8 mmol/l
IgG	less than 15% of total protein
Pressure	40–150 mm of CSF
Volume	c. 150 ml (adults)

Bromide partition test
Give intravenous sodium bromide 8.0 g in 30 ml, or oral 1.0 g t.i.d for three days. On the day after IV injection or end of oral intake obtain 5 ml venous blood and 3 ml CSF.

Normal ratio blood: CSF	2–3 : 1
Tuberculous meningitis	< 1.6 : 1

Respiratory function

Vital capacity	M 3.45–5.9 l
	F 2.45–4.4 l
Less than 1.0 l critical	
Arterial pH	38–44 nmol/l (7.33–7.45)
Arterial P_{CO_2}	5–6 kPa (37–45 mm Hg)
Arterial P_{O_2}	14 kPa (104 mm Hg)*

*varies with the O_2 concentration in inspired air

Urine

Sodium	60–350 mmol/24 h
Potassium	< 100 mmol/24 h
Calcium	2.5–7.5 mmol/24 h*
Vanillylmandelic acid (VMA)	< 35 µmol/24 h
5-Hydroxy-indoleacetic acid (5HIAA)	< 50 µmol/24 h
Protein	< 150 mg/24 h
Osmolality	430–1650 mosmol/24 h
maximal concentration	> 600 mosmol/kg

*affected by diet

REFERENCES

Hachinski, V. C., Iliff, L. D., Zilkha, E., du Boulay, G. H., McAllister, V. L., Marshall, J., Ross Russell, R. and Symon, L. (1975). *Archives of Neurology,* 32: 632.

Horowitz, S. H., Genkins, G., Kornfeld, P. and Papatestas, A. E. (1976). *Neurology,* 26: 410.

Hughes, R. A. C., Newsom-Davis, J. M., Perkin, G. D. and Pierce, J. (1978). *Lancet,* ii. 750.

Munzat, T. L. (1970). *Neurology,* 20: 1171.

Stevens, D. L. and Matthews, W. B. (1973). *British Medical Journal,* i: 439.

Teasdale, G. and Jennett, B. (1974). *Lancet,* ii: 81.

Thompson, E. J., Kaufmann, P., Shortman, R. C., Rudge, P. and McDonald, W. I. (1979). *British Medical Journal,* i: 16.

Till, K. (1975). *Paediatric Neurosurgery,* Oxford: Blackwell Scientific Publications.

Trimble, M. R. (1978). *British Medical Journal,* ii: 1682

Further Reading

Brooke, M. H. (1977). *A Clinician's View of Neuromuscular Diseases,* Baltimore: Williams & Wilkins.

Cogan, D. G. (1969). *Neurology of the Ocular Muscles,* Springfield: Charles C. Thomas.

Gordon, N. (1976). *Paediatric Neurology for the Clinician,* Clinics in Developmental Medicine 59/60, Spastics International Medical Publications, London: William Heinemann Medical Books.

Jennett, B. (1975). *Epilepsy after Non-Missile Head Injuries,* London: William Heinemann Medical Books.

Lishman, W. A. (1978). *Organic Psychiatry,* Oxford: Blackwell.

Marshall, J. (1976). *The Management of Cerebrovascular Disease,* Oxford: Blackwell.

Northfield, D. W. C. (1973). *The Surgery of the Central Nervous System,* Oxford: Blackwell.

Plum, F. and Posner, J. B. (1980). *Diagnosis of Stupor and Coma,* Philadelphia: F. A. Davis.

Till, K. (1975). *Paediatric Neurosurgery,* Oxford and London: Blackwell.

Walton, J. N. (1977). *Brain's Diseases of the Nervous System,* Oxford: Oxford University Press.

Wood, B. (1974). *A Paediatric Vade-Mecum,* London: Lloyd-Luke.

INDEX OF PROPRIETARY NAMES

Drug Proper Name	*Proprietary Name*
Acetazolamide	Diamox
Acycloguanosine	Acyclovir
Amantadine	Symmetrel
Aminocaproic acid	Epsikapron
Amphotericin B	Fungizone
Ampicillin	Penbritin
Azathioprine	Imuran
Baclofen	Lioresal
Benapryzine	Brizin
Benserazide + dopa	Madopar
Benzhexol	Artane
Benztropine	Cogentin
Bromocriptine	Parlodel
Carbamazepine	Tegretol
Carbidopa	Sinemet
Chloramphenicol	Chloromycetin
Chlormethiazole	Heminevrin
Chloroquine	Avloclor, Nivaquine
Cinnarizine	Stugeron
Clomipramine	Anafranil
Clonazepam	Rivotril
Clonidine	Dixarit
Dantrolene sodium	Dantrium
Dexamethasone	Decadron, Oradexon-Organon
Diazepam	Valium, Atensine
Diazoxide	Eudemine
Edrophonium	Tensilon
Erythromycin	Ilosone, Erythrocin
Ethambutol	Myambutol
Ethosuximide	Zarontin

Flucloxacillin	Floxapen
Flucytosine	Alcobon
Frusemide	Lasix
Gentamicin	Genticin
Glutethimide	Doriden
Haloperidol	Serenace
Hydralazine	Apresoline
Hydroxocobalamin	Neo-Cytamen
Imipramine	Tofranil
Iodophendylate	Myodil, Pantopaque
Isoniazid (INAH)	Rimifon
Lithium	Camcolit, Priadel
Methylphenidate	Ritalin
Methysergide	Deseril
Metoclopramide	Maxolon
Metrizamide	Amipaque
Metronidazole	Flagyl
Neostigmine	Prostigmin
Nitrazepam	Mogadon
Nitrofurantoin	Furadantin
Orphenadrine	Disipal
Pancuronium	Pavulon
Penicillamine	Distamine, Cuprimine
Phenobarbitone	Gardenal, Luminal
Phenoxybenzamine	Dibenyline
Phenytoin	Epanutin, Dilantin
Pizotifen	Sanomigran
Primidone	Mysoline
Procainamide	Pronestyl
Prochlorperazine	Stemetil, Vertigon
Procyclidine	Kemadrin

Propantheline	Probanthine
Propranolol	Inderal
Pyrazinamide	Zinamide
Pyridostigmine	Mestinon
Rifampicin	Rifadin
Sodium iothalamate	Conray
Sodium valproate	Epilim
Spironolactone	Aldactone
Tetrabenazine	Nitoman
Tetracycline	Achromycin
Thiopentone	Pentothal, Intraval Sodium
Thiopropazate	Dartalan
Tranexamic acid	Cyklokapron
Valproate	Epilim
Vincristine	Oncovin

INDEX

Abducens nerve (CN 6), 7
Abscess, cerebral, 49
Accessory nerve (CN 11), 11
Achondroplasia, 89
Acoustic neuroma, 83
Acromegaly, 81, 89
Action tremor, 104
Adenoma, pituitary, 80
Adie's pupil, tonic, 8
Adrenal deficiency, 123
Adversive seizures, 8, 79
Afferent pupillary defect, 6
Agnosia, 79
Akinetic fits, 63
Akinetic mutism, 31
Air-encephalography, 29
Alcoholism, 123
Alzheimer's disease, 98
Amaurosis fugax, 59
Amnesia, post traumatic, 129
   transient global, 68

Ampicillin, 46
Amyotrophic lateral sclerosis, 102
Anaemia, pernicious, 111
Anaesthesia, dissociated, 93
Anal reflex, 17
Aneurysm, rupture, 58
Angiography, 29
Angioma, 58, 83
Anosmia, 5
Anoxic coma, 35
Anterior inferior cerebellar artery
   syndrome, 55
Anticholinergic drugs, 106
Anticoagulants, 57, 61
Anticonvulsant drugs, side effects, 66
   therapeutic levels, 65
Antidiuretic hormone, 35, 112, 125
Apneustic breathing, 32
Apraxia, 79
Argyll Robertson pupil, 8
Arterial occlusion, 55

Arteritis, giant cell, 71
Ataxia, 16
Ataxic nystagmus, 9
Athetosis, 104
Atlanto-axial subluxation, 89
Auditory nerve (CN 8), 10
Auras, 79
Autonomic function, 17
Autonomic neuropathy, 110, 111

B_1 deficiency, 122
B_{12} deficiency, 111
Babinski reflex, 16
Bacterial infections, 44
Basal ganglia, 104
Basilar ischaemia, 59
Beri-beri, 122
Biochemical values, 135
Biopsy, brain, 51
  muscle, 115
  nerve, 113
Bladder, control, 17
  disturbance, 86
Blepharoclonus, 105
Blepharospasm, 105
Blood gases, 36
Blood viscosity, 57, 60
Bowel function, 17
Bradykinesia, 105
Brain stem, demyelination, 94
  infarction, 55
  tumour, 80
Breath holding attacks, 69
Broca's aphasia, 79
Bromide partition, 23, 46
Bromocriptine, 83, 107
Brown-Sequard syndrome, 86
Bulbar paralysis, 37

Calcification, intracranial, 27
Calcium, disturbances, 125
Caloric tests, 9, 10
Carbamazepine, 65, 66, 72, 96
Carbon dioxide tension, 36

Carcinomatous meningitis, 112
  non-metastatic complications, 128
  root compression, 92
Carotid artery TIAs, 59
Carotid sinus sensitivity, 67
Carpal tunnel syndrome, 110
Cataplexy, 68
Cauda equina claudicans, 88
Cavernous sinus thrombosis, 49, 97
Central neurogenic hyperventilation, 32
Cerebellar, astrocytoma, 81
  ataxia, 16, 76
  degeneration, 103
  tumours, 80
Cerebral, abscess, 49
  atrophy, 98
  dominance, 5
  embolism, 54
  haemorrhage, 54
  metastases, 83
  oedema, 57, 84
  thrombosis, 55
  tumours, 76
Cerebrospinal fluid, bromide partition, 23
  gamma globulin, 95
  lactate, 23
  leaks, 132
  meningitis, 45, 46
  normal values, 136
Cerebrospinal syphilis, 52
Cerebrovascular disease, 54
Cervical myelopathy, 90
  radiculopathy, 90
  spondylosis, 90
Charcot joints, 53
Charcot-Marie-Tooth disease, 103
Cheyne Stokes respiration, 31, 35
Chiasmal compression, 82
Chloramphenicol, 45, 46
Cholinergic crisis, 42, 121
Chorda tympani, 9
Chorea, Huntington's, 100, 104
  'pill' induced, 108
  pregnancy, 108
  Sydenham's, 107
Chromophobe adenoma, 80
Cisternal puncture, 23
Clonazepam, 43, 108
Clonus, 12
Cloward's procedure, 91

Coma, causes, 31, 33, 34
  investigation, 35
  scale, 4
  treatment, 36
Communicating hydrocephalus, 101
Confusion, 31
Conjugate eye movements, 8
Connective tissue disorders, 126
Conn's syndrome, 125
Consciousness, transient loss of, causes, 67
Continuing stroke, 54
Convulsions, febrile, 63
Co-ordination, 16
Copper, in Wilson's disease, 107
Corneal reflex, 9
Cortisol, 22
Cough syncope, 67
Cranial arteritis, 71
Cranial nerves, 5
Creatine phosphokinase, 22, 115
Cremasteric reflex, 16
Cushing's syndrome, 81, 123
Cutaneous nerve distribution, 18, 19

Deafness, 10
Decerebrate rigidity, 33
Decorticate rigidity, 33
Dejerine-Sottas disease, 103
Delerium, 31
Delerium tremens, 123
Dementia, causes, 98, 99
  investigations of, 98
  multi-infarct, 101
Demyelinating disease, 93
  CSF in, 95
  electrophysiological studies, 95
  treatment of, 96
Depressive headache, 73
Dermatomes, 18, 19
Devic's disease, 97
Dexamethasone 57, 85
Dextran-40, 57
Diabetes insipidus, 22, 81
Diabetes mellitus, 111
Diabetic, amyotrophy, 92
  coma,
    hyperosmolar, 34
    hypoglycaemic, 33
    ketotic, 34
  neuropathy, 111
Dialysis dementia, 125
Diazepam, in, spasticity, 96
  status epilepticus, 43
  tetanus, 40
Diplopia, assessment, 8
Discs, prolapsed intervertebral, 89
Disseminated intravascular coagulopathy, 45
Disseminated sclerosis, *see* Multiple sclerosis, 93
Dissociated sensory loss, 93
Disturbed patients, 3
Doll's head manoeuvres, 32
Dopa, 106
Dopamine, 106
Drop attacks, basilar ischaemia, in, 59
  cryptogenic, 68
Drowsiness, 31
Duchenne dystrophy, 116
Dysarthria, 59, 80, 95
Dyscalculia, 5
Dysconjugate eye movements, 32
Dysgraphia, 5
Dyslexia, 5
Dysphasia, 5
Dystonia, 104
Dystrophia myotonica, 117
Dystrophies,
  see Muscular dystrophies, 116

Eaton-Lambert syndrome, 128
Echo-encephalography, 29
Edrophonium (Tensilon) test, 42, 120
Electrocardiography, 24
Electroencephalography, 24
Electrolyte disturbances, 125
Electromyography, 24
Electronystagmography, 25
Embolism, 54
Empty sella, 82
Empyema, subdural, 49
Encephalitis, 50
  causes of, 48

herpes simplex, 50
SSPE, 100
viral, 50
Encephalopathy, hypertensive, 61
progressive multifocal, 128
Wernicke's, 122
Endocrine glands,
adrenal, 22, 123
muscle disorders, 119
normal values, 136
pituitary function tests, 21
thyroid, 21
Ependymoma, 82
Epilepsy, 62
causes, 64
childhood, 63
focal, 63
grand mal, tonic/clonic, 62
investigation of, 64
minor, 63
myoclonic, 63
petit mal, 63
post-traumatic, 132
status epilepticus, 43
temporal lobe, 62
treatment of, 65
tumours, 77
Erb's spastic paraplegia, 53
Ergotamine, 70
Ethambutol, 47
Ethosuximide, 65, 66
Evoked potentials, 25
Exophthalmic ophthalmoplegia, 119
Extradural haematoma, 131
Extrapyramidal disorders, 104
Eye movements, in unconscious patients, 32
testing, 8
volitional control of, 8

Facial nerve (CN 7), 9
Facio-scapulo-humeral dystrophy, 117
Faints, syncope, 67
False localising signs, 77
Familial periodic paralysis, 125
Febrile convulsions, 63
Femoral neuropathy, 92

Femoral stretch test, 89
Fits, see epilepsy, 62
Fluorescein angiography, 25
Focal fits, 63
Folate deficiency, 122
Foraminal cone, 78
Friedreich's ataxia, 102
Frontal lobe signs, 79
Frusemide, 57
Fungal infections, 48

Gag reflex, 11, 32
Gait, 16
General paralysis of the insane (GPI), 53
Geniculate zoster, 51
Giant cell arteritis, 71
Giddiness, 73
Glabellar tap, 9
Glasgow coma scale, 3, 4
Gliomas, 82
Glossopharyngeal nerve (CN 9), 11
Glossopharyngeal neuralgia, 72
Glycerol, 57
Grand mal fits, 62
Grasp reflex, 79
Guillain-Barré syndrome, 39
Gumma, 53

Haemangioblastoma, 83
Haematological values, 135
Haemorrhage, subarachnoid, 58
Haemorrhagic infarction, 54
Headache, 69
acute, 69
chronic, 73
cluster, 70
depressive, 73
elevated intracranial pressure, 71
investigation, 73
migrainous, 69
post-lumbar-puncture, 71
tension, 73
Head injuries, 129
acute haematomata, 130

cerebral oedema, 132
management of, 129
medico-legal considerations, 133
sequelae, 132
Hearing testing, 10
Hemianopia, 7
Hemiballismus, 104
Hemiplegic migraine, 69
Hepatic failure, 124
Herpes simplex encephalitis, 50
Herpes zoster, 51
complications of, 51
Herxheimer reaction, 53
Hormones, 21
Horner's syndrome, 8
Huntington's chorea, 100
Hydrocephalus, communicating, 101
obstructive, 67, 77, 80
Hyperaldosteronism, 125
Hypercalcaemia, 126
Hypertension, 57, 61
Hypertensive encephalopathy, 61
Hyperventilation, 68
Hypnagogic hallucinations, 68
Hypocalcaemia, 68, 125
Hypoglossal nerve, (CN 12), 11
Hypoglycaemia, 33, 68
Hypokalaemia, 125
Hyponatraemia, 125
Hypopituitary function, 21, 80
Hypothalamic symptoms, 80
Hypsarrhythmia, 63
Hysterical fits, 68

Imbalance, 75
Inappropriate secretion of antidiuretic hormone, 112, 125, 130
Incontinence, 20
Incoordination, 16, 86, 95
Infantile spasms, 63
Infarction, cerebral 54, 55
Infection, bacterial, 44
meningitic, 44
syphilitic, 52
tuberculous, 46
viral, 47
Innervation of muscles, 14, 15

Intelligence tests, 4, 5
Intention tremor, 80, 104
Internuclear ophthalmoplegia, 8
Intervertebral disc prolapse, 89
Intracranial pressure, elevated, 77
headache with, 71
symptoms of elevated, 77
reduction of, 84
Involuntary movements, 104
Ischaemia, transient cerebral, 54, 59
Ischaemic score, 101
Isoniazid, 47

Jacksonian epilepsy, 62, 63
Jakob-Creutzfeldt disease, 100
Jarisch-Herxheimer reaction, 53
Jaw jerk, 12, 16
Jerks, tendon, 13

Kayser-Fleischer ring, 107
Kernig's sign, 33, 44
Ketotic diabetic coma, 34
Korsakoff syndrome, 122

Lactate, CSF, 23
Laminectomy, 91
Landry-Guillain-Barré syndrome, 39
Lateral popliteal nerve compression, 111
Leptospiral meningitis, 48
Lhermitte's phenomenon, 86, 94
Lightning pains, 53
Limb-girdle dystrophy, 116
Liver failure, 35, 124
Liver function tests, 22
Locked-in syndrome, 31
Locomotor ataxia, 53
Lower motor neurone features, 12
Lumbar puncture, 22
Lumbar spondylosis, 89
Lymphoma, 113, 128

Major fits, tonic/clonic, 62
Malabsorption, 122
Manipulation, spinal, 91
Mannitol, 57, 84
Marche à petits pas, 16
Median longitudinal fasciculus, 8
Median nerve compression, 110
Medulloblastoma, 81
Memory, assessment, 4, 5
Menière's disease, 74
Meningioma, 82
Meningism, 33, 44
Meningitis, 44
  bacterial, 45
  carcinomatous, 112
  diagnosis of, 44
  fungal, 48
  haemophilus, 46
  leptospiral, 48
  meningococcal, 45
  partially treated, 49
  pneumococcal, 46
  symptoms of, 44
  syphilitic, 52
  treatment of, 45
  tuberculous, 46
  viral, 47
Meningovascular syphilis, 52
Metastases, cerebral, 83
Metrizamide, 30
Micturition syncope, 67
Migraine, 69
  basilar, 67, 69
  loss of consciousness in, 67
  ophthalmoplegic, 70
  treatment of, 70
Migrainous neuralgia, 70
Mononeuritis multiplex, 111
Motor function, assessment, 12
Motor neurone disease, 101
Multiple sclerosis, 93
  CSF in, 95
  diagnosis of, 95
  optic neuritis, 95
  paroxysmal disorders, 95
  presentation of, 94
  treatment of, 96
Mumps, 47, 48
Muscle disease, 114
  biopsy, 115
  carrier detection, 116
  endocrine disorders, 119
  inflammatory, 118
  investigation, 115
  polymyositis, 118
  thyrotoxic, 119
Muscle innervation, 14, 15
Muscle power, 12
Muscular dystrophies, 116
  Duchenne, 116
  facio-scapulo-humeral, 117
  limb girdle, 116
  myotonic, 117
  ocular, 117
Myasthenia gravis, 42, 119
  antibodies in, 120
  cholinergic crisis, 42
  diagnosis, 120
  edrophonium test, 42, 120
  myasthenic crisis, 42
  presentation of, 119
  thymectomy, 121
  treatment of, 120
Myelitis, 97
Myelography, 29
Myelopathy, spondylotic, 90
Myoclonic fits, 63
Myoclonus, 108
  anoxic, 35
Myodil, 30
Myotomes, 13, 14, 15
Myotonia, 117
Myxoedema, 76, 111

Narcolepsy, 68
Neonatal fits, 63, 64
Neonatal meningitis, 45
Neostigmine, 42, 121,
Nerve,
  abducens (CN 6), 7
  accessory (CN 11), 11
  auditory (CN 8), 10
  biopsy, 113
  conduction, 113
  facial, (CN 7), 9
  glossopharyngeal (CN 9), 11
  hypoglossal (CN 12), 11
  lateral popliteal, 111
  median, 110

oculomotor, (CN 3), 7
olfactory (CN 1), 5
optic, (CN 2), 6
  roots,
  dermatomes, 18, 19
  myotomes, 13, 14, 15
trigeminal (CN 5), 9
trochlear, (CN 4), 7
ulnar, 111
vagal, (CN 10), 11
Neuralgia, migrainous, 70
  glossopharyngeal, 72
  post herpetic, 51
  trigeminal, 72
Neuralgic amyotrophy, 92
Neuroma, acoustic, 83
Neuromyelitis optica, 97
Neuronitis, vestibular, 74
Neuropathic joints, 53, 93
Neuropathy, 108
  acute, 39
  alcoholic, 123
  B_1 deficiency, 112
  B_{12} deficiency, 111
  carcinomatous, 112
  causes of, 109
  diabetic, 111
  entrapment, 110
  femoral, 92
  Guillain-Barré, 39
  investigation of, 113
  porphyria, 112
  senile, 110
  uraemic, 124
Neurosyphilis, 52
Nominal dysphasia, 5
Non-metastatic complications of malignancy, 128
Nystagmus, 9
  ataxic, 9
  central, 9
  cerebellar, 75, 80
  optokinetic, 6
  peripheral, 9
  positional, 11

Obstructive hydrocephalus, 67
Occipital lobe signs, 80

Ocular movements, 8
Ocular myopathy, 117
Oculo-cephalic reflexes, 32
Oculomotor nerve (CN 3) 7
Oculo-vestibular reflexes, 10, 32
Oedema, cerebral, 57
Olfactory nerve, (CN 1), 5
Ophthalmic zoster, 51
Ophthalmoplegia, internuclear, 8
Opisthotonus, 40
Optic atrophy, 6, 95
Optic chiasm, 7
Optic disc, 6
Optic nerve (CN 2), 6
Optic neuritis, 95
Optic radiation, 7
Optic tract, 7
Optokinetic nystagmus, 6
Osmolality, 22
Otolith, 11
Oxygen tension, 36

Paget's disease, 89
Palsy, bulbar, 37
Panencephalitis, subacute sclerosing, 100
Papillitis, 95
Papilloedema, 6
Paralysis, bulbar, 37
  respiratory, 37
Paraplegia, 85
Parasagittal meningioma, 82
Parkinson's disease, 105
  treatment, 106
Parietal lobe symptoms, 79
Parinaud's syndrome, 8
Penicillin,
  in meningitis, 45
  in syphilis, 52
Perimetry, 6
Perineal sensation, 17
Periodic paralysis, 125
Peripheral neuropathy,
  see neuropathy, 108
Pernicious anaemia, 111
Peroneal muscular atrophy, 103
Perseveration, 5
Petit mal, 63
Phenobarbitone, 65, 66

Phenytoin, 65, 66
Pheochromocytoma, 123
Phytanic acid, 103
Pituitary, apoplexy, 83
   function tests, 21
   tumours, 82
   treatment, 83
Plantar response, 16
Pneumo-encephalography, 29
Poliomyelitis, 41
Polyarteritis nodosa (PAN) 126
Polymyalgia rheumatica, 118
Polymyositis, 118
Polyneuritis *see* neuropathy, 108
Porphyria, 112
Post-concussive syndrome, 133
Posterior column sensation, 17
Posterior fossa symptoms, 80
Posterior inferior cerebellar artery syndrome, 55
Post-herpetic neuralgia, 51
Post-traumatic amnesia, 129
Post-traumatic epilepsy, 132
Potassium disturbances, 125
Presenile dementia, 98
Pressure cones, 78
Pressure palsies, 110
Primidone, 65, 66
Progressive, bulbar palsy, 102
   multifocal leuco-encephalopathy, 128
   muscular atrophy, 102
   supranuclear palsy, 107
Prolactin secreting tumours, 81
Prolactin test in fits, 69
Prolapsed intervertebral discs, 89
   investigation of, 90
   treatment of, 91
Protein in CSF, 136
   in meningitis, 45
   in multiple sclerosis, 95
Pseudo-athetosis, 86
Psychometric tests, 5
Ptosis, 8
Pupils, Adie (tonic), 8
   afferent defect, 6
   Argyll Robertson, 8
   fixed, 32
   in coma, 32
   light-near dissociation, 8
   pin-point, 32

Pyrazinamide, 47
Pyridostigmine, 121

Queckenstedt's test, 23, 88

Radiological tests, 26
Radiotherapy, in cerebral tumours, 82, 83
Ramsay Hunt syndrome, 51
Red cell transketolase, 22
Reflexes, abdominal, 16
   anal, 17
   Babinski, 16
   corneal, 9, 32
   cremasteric, 16
   facial, 9
   gag, 11, 32
   superficial, 16
   tendon, 13
Refsum's disease, 103
Renal failure, 124
Respiratory failure, 36
   treatment, 38
Respiratory function, 37
   normal values, 137
Retinal photography, 25
Rheumatoid arthritis, 126
Rifampicin, 47
Rigidity, decerebrate, 33
   decorticate, 33
   Parkinsonian, 105
RIHSA scans, 28
Rinne's test, 10
Romberg's sign, 16
Root tension signs, 89

Salaam attacks, 63
Sarcoidosis, 127
Scans, CT, 28
   isotope, 28
   RIHSA, 28, 101
Self poisoning, 33
Sensation,
   dermatomes, 18, 19
   testing, 17

Sensory ataxia, 76
Shingles (zoster), 51
Sleep paralysis, 68
Smell, test, 5
Spasmodic torticollis, 105
Spasticity, 96
Speech upsets, 5, 79
Sphenopalatine, neuralgia, 70
Sphincter upset due to cord compression, 86
Spinal cord compression, 85
  causes of, 85
  investigation of, 88
  presentation of, 86
  treatment of, 88
Spinal degenerative disease, 89
  cervical, 90
  lumbar, 89
  treatment of, 91
Spinal tumours, 85
Spino-cerebellar degeneration, 76, 102
Spinothalamic tract, 17
Status epilepticus, 43
Steele-Richardson-Olszewski's syndrome, 107
Streptomycin, 47
Stroke, acute, 54
  in evolution, 54
  investigations, 56
  management of, 55
  mortality, 58
  risks, 61
  treatment of, 56
Stupor, 31
Subacute combined degeneration of the spinal cord, 111
Subacute sclerosing panencephalitis, 100
Subarachnoid haemorrhage, 58, 70
  treatment of, 59
Subclavian steal, 60
Subdural empyema, 49
Subdural haematoma, 72, 131
Substantia nigra, 104
Subthalamic nucleus, 104
Sulphonamides, 45
Superior cerebellar artery syndrome, 55
Swallowing, 37
Sweating, 20
Sydenham's chorea, 107
Sympathetic ocular paresis, 8

Sympathetic upset in tetanus, 40
Syncope, 67
  cough-, 67
  micturition-, 67
Syphilis, 52
Syringobulbia, 92
Syringomyelia, 92
Systemic lupus erythematosus (SLE), 126

Tabes dorsalis, 53
Taboparesis, 53
Taste, 10
Temporal arteritis, 71
Temporal lobe epilepsy, 62
Temporal lobe symptoms 79
Tendon reflexes, 12
Tensilon (endrophonium) test, 42, 120
Tension headache, 73
Tentorial herniation, 78
Tetanus, 40
Tetany, 68, 125
Thiamine deficiency, 35, 122
Thomsen's disease, 117
Thrombophlebitis, intracranial, 49
Thrombotic infarction, 55
Thymectomy, 121
Thymoma, 120
Thyroid function, 21
Thyrotoxic, myopathy, 119
  opthalmoplegia, 119
Tone, muscle, 12
Tonic/clonic fits, 62
Tonic pupil (Adie), 8
Torsion dystonia, 104
Traction, spinal, 91
Tracheostomy, 38
Transient amaurosis, 59
Transient global amnesia, 68
Transient ischaemic attacks, 54, 59
  precipitants, 60
  treatment of, 61
Transient loss of consciousness, causes of, 67
Transient visual obscurations, 71, 78
Trauma, *see* head injuries, 129
Traumatic CSF tap, 23

Tremor, 104
  essential, 105
  familial, 105
  intention, 80, 104,
  Parkinsonian, 105
  positional, 104
  senile, 104
Trigeminal nerve (CN 5), 9
Trigeminal neuralgia, 72, 95
Triple bolus test, pituitary, 21
Trismus, 40
Trochlear nerve (CN 4), 7
Tuberose sclerosis, 64, 99
Tuberculous meningitis, 46
Tumours, cerebral, 76
  adults, 77, 82
  children, 77, 81
  frontal lobe, 79
  investigation of, 84
  occipital lobe, 80
  parietal lobe, 79
  posterior fossa, 80
  temporal lobe, 79

Ulnar nerve palsy, 111
Unconscious patients, 30
  investigation of, 35
  treatment of, 36
Unsteadiness, chronic, 75
Upper motor neurone signs, 12
Uraemia, 124
Urine, normal values, 137
Useless hand, 94

Vagus nerve (CN 10), 11
Valproate sodium, 65, 66
Vascular disorders, 54
Vegetative state, 31
Venous sinus thrombosis, 49
Ventilation, artificial, 38
Ventriculo-atrial shunt, 85
Ventriculography, 30
Ventriculo-peritoneal shunt, 85
Vertebrobasilar ischaemia, 59

Vertigo, 73
  benign paroxysmal, 69
  benign positional, 11, 74
  causes of, 75
  investigation of, 76
  tests, 11
Vestibular function, 10
Vestibular neuronitis, 74
Vidian neuralgia, 70
Viral infections, 47
Visual acuity, 6
Visual evoked responses, 25
Visual fields, 7
Visual loss, acute, 97
Visual obscurations, 71, 78
Vital capacity, 37, 137
Vitamin deficiency, B_1, 122
  B_{12}, 111
  others, 122
Voice, hoarse, 11
Vomiting, elevated intracranial pressure, 77
Von Hippel Lindau's disease, 84

Wassermann reaction and serological tests for syphilis, 52
Waterhouse-Friderichsen's syndrome, 45
Water intoxication, 125
Weber's test, 10
Wechsler adult intelligence scale (WAIS), 5
Wegener's granuloma, 127
Wernicke-Korsakoff syndrome, 122
West's syndrome, 63
Wilson's disease, 107
Withdrawal fits, 64
Withdrawal states, alcoholic, 123

Xanthochromic CSF, 23
X-rays, chest, 27
  pineal, 27
  pituitary fossa, 27
  skull, 26
  special, 28
  spinal, 27